Understanding Anemia

Understanding Health and Sickness Series
Miriam Bloom, Ph.D.
General Editor

Understanding Anemia

Ed Uthman, M.D.

University Press of Mississippi
Jackson

OI OO 99 98   4 3 2 I
The paper in this book meets the guidelines for permanence and durability
of the Committee on Production Guidelines for Book Longevity of the
Council on Library Resources.

Library of Congress Cataloging-in-Publication Data

Uthman, Ed
     Understanding anemia / Ed Uthman.
          p.   cm.—(Understanding health and sickness series)
     Includes bibliographical references and index.
          ISBN 1-57806-038-9 (cloth : alk. paper).—ISBN 1-57806-039-7
     (pbk. : alk. paper)
          I. Anemia—Popular works.   I. Title.   II. Series.
     RC641.U87   1998
     616.1'52—dc21   97-29076
                                                                    CIP

British Library Cataloging-in-Publication data available

Contents

Acknowledgments and Dedication

Much of my gratitude for help with this book goes to those hematologists and hematopathologists who years ago taught me the basics of blood: Lemuel Diggs, Marion Dugdale, Carolyn Chesney, Charles Neely, John Shively, and Frank White. Nonphysician professionals involved in my training to whom I am no less grateful are James Mason, Ann Bell, Helen Goodman, and Pam Turpin.

In more recent years, I have benefited from the knowledgeable comments of my highly valued physician colleagues, and each of these contributed knowingly or unknowingly to this book: Luther Burkett, William Grunow, Royce Joyner, Elizabeth Hartwell, Charles Conlon, and Charles Crumb. And, of course, there is my favorite physician, Margaret Uthman, to whom I am doubly indebted.

I would like to express posthumous thanks to Isaac Asimov, whose books I have read from childhood on, and whose clarity of language and enthusiasm for knowledge will be forever worthy of emulation.

While this book would not exist without the collective contribution of the people mentioned above, all opinions and errors here are ultimately mine.

This book is dedicated to Margaret, Riss, and Drew.

Introduction

Anemia is one of the most common conditions encountered in medical practice, yet it is poorly understood by the general public and can even give experienced doctors problems. Individuals who are victims of serious diseases typically experience anemia at some point in the course of their illness. Others suffer from anemia and live long healthy lives, never knowing of their condition. While anemia may strike at any age, some people are born with it and must deal with its complications for life. Some anemias are severe, incurable, and life-shortening, while others are either inconsequential or respond readily to treatment. Treatment of anemia can be as simple as improving one's diet or as complicated as performing a bone marrow transplant.

The purpose of this book is to introduce the reader to anemia—its classifications, causes, and treatments. The reader will learn that the various types of anemias are caused by different disturbances of physiology, and that ultimately there is a fundamental molecular basis for each. Every rare and esoteric anemia cannot be included here, but the common ones, which account for the overwhelming majority of cases of anemia, will be discussed in detail.

The book begins with a brief discussion of the history of the study of blood, then covers the fundamental anatomy and physiology of the blood and blood-forming tissues. We will see what anemia does to the body and how doctors make a diagnosis. The role of routine lab tests is discussed and a simple method of classifying anemias into three broad categories described. We will examine the individual anemias—first those caused by deficiency of nutrients, then those resulting from excess destruction of blood cells. We will also look at the important hereditary forms of anemia and, finally, several miscellaneous conditions.

This book is for the general reader with no medical training. It presumes a basic knowledge of biology at the high school level; for those who may feel a little rusty in that area, a quick review of cell biology is presented in appendix B. This book uses the metric system of measurement, which some find off-putting, but the brief explanation in appendix A should ameliorate any antipathy toward meters and liters.

I assume that most people will read this book to learn more about a case of anemia that has affected them personally. Although it is about blood, the book makes liberal detours into the nooks and crannies of nutrition, biochemistry, genetics, the digestive system, and the circulatory system. My hope is that some readers will follow this seductive, serpentine path into the fascinating world of medical science and find that it is one from which they do not wish to escape.

Understanding Anemia

1. What Is Anemia?

The word "anemia" is composed of two Greek roots that together mean "without blood," but to use this literal translation as a definition would be a gross exaggeration. Still, the modern definition is simple: *anemia is any condition characterized by an abnormal decrease in the body's total red blood cell mass.* To understand the definition, one has to understand what red blood cells are and what they do, how the body reacts to an abnormally low red cell mass, and what happens when the mass of red cells falls so low that the body cannot adapt to it. We will discuss these matters in this chapter, but first we will look at the history of anemia and its study.

HISTORICAL PERSPECTIVE

The ancients readily recognized the importance of blood as a life-giving substance, believing it to hold the body's vital force. Hebrews back to the patriarchal age maintained that blood was the seat of the soul and demanded through the Mosaic Laws that it be drained before an animal was prepared as food (a practice still followed by Orthodox Jews today). The Romans drank the blood of their enemies, thinking it would confer on them the courage of their vanquished foes. While today the concept of the circulation of the blood seems obvious, it was not until the relatively recent era of the seventeenth century that William Harvey determined that blood was not just a contained static liquid like hydraulic fluid.

The scientific study of blood had to await the invention of the microscope. While magnifying lenses were known to the monastic scholar and natural historian Roger Bacon (1214–94), lenses of sufficient quality for scientific use were not available for another three centuries. The first compound microscope (the great-granddaddy of the clinical microscope of today) was made in 1590 by the Dutch spectacle maker Zacharias Janssen. No one thought to use this instrument to look at blood until the noted Dutch naturalist Jan Swammerdam (1637–80), turned his instrument on the fluid of life and discovered what he called "ruddy globules," which were presumably red blood cells. The first detailed description of the red cells was produced by the famous (also Dutch) microscopist Antonj van Leeuwenhoek (1632–1723). While these men were great "natural historians," they were not medical researchers in the modern sense of the word. In fact, neither they nor those who immediately followed them thought that red cells were of any importance to the body. This realization had to await the insight of an Englishman, William Hewson (1739–74), whose posthumously published opinion that because red cells were present in such abundance they *had* to be important earned him the title "the father of hematology."

At the beginning of the nineteenth century, the word "anemia" was a clinical term referring to pallor of the skin and mucous membranes (the thin linings that cover the inside of the mouth, the whites of the eyes, the inner surface of the eyelids, and other surfaces not covered by skin). At the time of the publication of the first textbook of hematology by the French physician Gabriel Andral in 1843, there was no appreciation for the basic concept held today that clinical anemia is due to inadequate numbers of red blood cells. Before this could be determined, it was necessary to develop a technical method by which blood cells could be counted. This was first done in 1852 by Karl Vierordt, but his technique was too tedious to gain widespread use. Vierordt's student, H. Welcher, counted the cells in a patient with chlorosis (an old word for what is probably our modern iron-deficiency anemia) and found in 1854 that an anemic patient had significantly fewer red blood cells than a normal person. Thus, almost two centuries passed after Swammerdam's discovery of red cells in 1658 before it was shown that a deficiency in the number of red cells was behind the clinical diagnosis of anemia.

The clinical and biological science of hematology was given a tremendous boost in the period between 1878 and 1888, when it became possible to examine the microscopic details of blood cells. Interestingly, the event that provided this opportunity was not the development of the microscope, which was already fairly advanced by that time, but of biological stains. Although the human body is opaque and colorful to the naked eye, at the microscopic level almost all cells are nearly transparent. Most cells are completely colorless, and even those that have their own native color, like red blood cells, appear extremely pale and washed-out when viewed individually. Accordingly, few cellular details can be distinguished by looking at unstained specimens with even the best modern microscopes. It is necessary to stain the cells with dyes to obtain much useful information from them. The preeminent figure in the world of biological stains was Paul Ehrlich (1854–1915), the Silesian-born son of affluent Jewish parents and one of the truly great names in the history of biomedical science.

Ehrlich had done poorly in school as a boy, but he had shown great aptitude for and interest in biology and chemistry. His first major discovery was a good method for staining the bacterium that causes tuberculosis, which made the microscopic diagnosis of that important disease much easier. Unfortunately, he caught a mild case of it and had to take time off to recover. Ehrlich later worked out the details of preparing an antitoxin for another dreaded disease, diphtheria, which represented the first use of immunotherapy to specifically treat an infection (vaccines are also immunotherapy and had been around for much longer, but they prevent infections rather than treat them). Ehrlich's contribution won for his boss, Emil von Behring, the first Nobel Prize for physiology or medicine in 1901. Although Ehrlich had probably done most of the actual work, von Behring was given full credit for the discovery (Ehrlich eventually did get a Nobel in 1908 for other work).

Continuing to be interested in dyes, Ehrlich realized that something about their chemical makeup allowed them to attach themselves to specific parts of a cell. Combining this property with a poisonous one, he reasoned, should make it possible to create a dye-like substance that would attach itself to a specific infection-causing microorganism and kill it. This concept led Ehrlich to develop trypan red, a dye used in the treatment of trypanosomiasis (a class of parasitic infestations that includes African sleeping sickness), and arsphenamine, which was the first effective treatment for syphilis, another major public health problem of Victorian times.

Ehrlich's contribution to routine hematology was his development of the triacid stain, which allowed him to properly classify white blood cells into a scheme similar to the one used today. In 1891, the triacid stain was replaced by the eosin methylene blue stain invented by D. L. Romanowsky of St. Petersburg, Russia. The "Romanowsky stain" was further modified by Richard May of Munich in 1902, Gustav Giemsa of Hamburg in 1905, and J. H. Wright of Boston in 1906. All of these modifications were direct descendants of Ehrlich's original ideas. Over ninety years later, we still use two of these, the May-Gruenwald-Giemsa stain and the Wright stain, for the examination of the myriad blood smears routinely prepared in clinical laboratories every day.

Standing on the broad shoulders of nineteenth century giants like Ehrlich, twentieth century hematologists led their science at an ever-accelerating rate into the modern age, providing scientific explanations for the various types of anemia discussed in this book. Ever easier, faster, and cheaper ways to diagnose and classify anemias were developed, and techniques for treating them, from nutritional therapy to blood transfusion to bone marrow transplants, were devised. The era of modern hematology is considered to have begun at Harvard Medical School with the work of George Richards Minot (1885–1950) and his assistant, William Parry Murphy (1892–1987), who, between 1924 and 1926, found that patients who suffered from pernicious anemia could be successfully treated with large quantities of raw liver in their diets. Minot and Murphy shared the 1934 Nobel Prize for their discovery. From this point on, the investigation of anemia revolved around phenomena at the molecular level, which is where we are today.

BLOOD

Given the amount that flows from even a trivial cut, it is tempting to assume that the body is literally full of blood. Actually, blood makes up a small fraction of the body's volume. Consider an "average" man weighing 70 kilograms, or 154 pounds. Since the human body has just about the same density as water, and 1 liter of water weighs 1 kilogram, the total volume of his body is about 70 liters. Of this, only about 5 liters represents the total volume of blood. Therefore, blood accounts for only 7 percent of the total body volume. In the normal state, blood must stay confined to several anatomic structures meant to hold it. The first of these is the *circulatory system*, which consists of the heart and blood vessels. The heart's main function is to be a pump for the blood (although it has a lesser-known function in the endocrine system concerning the regulation of body water content and blood volume). The blood vessels consist of (1) *arteries*, thick-walled elastic structures that withstand the high pressures generated by the pumping action of the heart, (2) *veins*, thin-walled low-pressure vessels that conduct blood back to the heart, and (3) *capillaries*, microscopic tubes that ramify throughout all the tissues of the body (except the cartilage of the skeletal system and cornea of the eye, which are able to live without a direct blood supply). Arteries conduct blood from the heart to innumerable beds of capillaries, which have such thin walls that exchange of nutrients, hormones, and waste products between the blood and tissues is easily accomplished. The capillaries converge into small veins, which converge into larger veins to conduct the blood back to the heart under very low pressure, where the pumping cycle begins again. The heart actually consists of two separate pumps in series; these just happen to be stuck to each other side by side. The right heart collects oxygen-poor blood, which has a dark purple color, from veins arriving from all the tissues of the body and pumps it into the lungs, where inhaled oxygen is picked up and carbon dioxide is dropped off to be exhaled. The oxygen-rich blood, which is bright red, is returned to the left heart and pumped out to the periphery of the body to complete the cycle.

The other anatomic structure for containing the blood is the *reticuloendothelial system* (RES), which consists of cavern-like structures called *sinusoids* lying within the spleen, liver, and bone marrow. The function of the sinusoids is to facilitate the exposure of blood to certain cells that are involved in the immune response to foreign invaders. Sinusoids in the bone marrow also serve as embarkation areas for newly born blood cells beginning their journey in the circulation. Blood flow through the sinusoids is very slow, so as to allow the blood maximum contact time with the tissues charged with these complex interactions.

Blood in a test tube would appear to be an inert liquid, but it is in fact no less a living, breathing tissue than is the heart, brain, or any other body part. Physically, blood consists of cells suspended in a liquid medium. The liquid medium, accounting for about 60 percent of the volume of blood, is called *plasma*. Of the plasma, about 93 percent is water. The remainder consists of suspended and dissolved solids, the most abundant of which is a protein called *albumin*. Other proteins in the plasma are called *globulins*. Both types of proteins have a variety of functions, some of which will be discussed later. There is also a set of important proteins in the plasma involved in the coagulation of the blood; these are called, appropriately enough, *coagulation factors*. If you take plasma from the blood and allow it to coagulate (form a clot), the resulting fluid left after the clot is removed is called *serum*. Several of the important laboratory measurements employed in the evaluation of anemias involve the determination of the quantity of nutrients and other substances in serum. These will also be discussed later.

BLOOD CELLS

The cells of the blood constitute about 40 percent of its volume. Of this volume, the overwhelming proportion is represented by the *red blood cells* (RBCs), or *erythrocytes*. There are about 5 million RBCs in every microliter of blood. Since there are about 5 million microliters of blood in the body (5 liters times 1 million microliters per liter), there are approximately 5 million times 5 million, or 25 trillion, red cells present. The whole body has an estimated 50 trillion cells of all types; thus, red blood cells account for about half the cells in the body. It may seem surprising that half of the body's cells are confined to 7 percent of its volume, until one considers how small and packed together the red cells are compared to the others. In fact, the red cell is smaller than just about any cell in the body, the sperm being a rather memorable exception.

Red cells, like most blood cells, are made in the *bone marrow*, the spongy internal core of most bones. In children the entire skeleton contains hematopoietic (blood cell-producing) marrow, but, as we age, marrow cell production becomes confined to bones in the central portion of the body, namely those of the spinal column, pelvis, skull, sternum (breastbone), hip and shoulder. In the adult, the weight of active marrow is about 4½ pounds, making the marrow the second largest organ in the body (after the skin). Red cells begin their existence as marrow cells called *erythroblasts* (in biological parlance, a "blast" is a primitive cell from which other, more mature, cells form). These cells have nuclei with DNA and can reproduce themselves like the many other self-replicating cells in the body. Some of the erythroblasts reach a point at which they stop reproducing themselves and instead go out into the wide world of the bloodstream as erythrocytes. To do this they have to spend several days in the marrow undergoing a sequence of events called maturation, by which they (1) become progressively more filled with hemoglobin, and (2) eventually lose their nuclei. The resulting cell is essentially a sac containing hemoglobin and the biochemical minifactory necessary to maintain the chemical integrity of hemoglobin. The shape of the red cell is referred to as a biconcave disc. (A donut with its hole partially filled in is a good analogy.) It is essential that the red cell maintain its normal biconcave disc shape; otherwise, it is quickly destroyed by various police cells in the reticuloendothelial system.

After release into the bloodstream, red cells circulate for an average lifespan of 120 days. Therefore, every day, $\frac{1}{120}$ of the total erythrocyte mass must be replaced. This comes out to 200 billion red cells per day, or over 2 million per second. If that's not enough of a task, the marrow must also produce most of the other types of cells in the blood.

The other cellular constituents of the blood are the *white cells* (leukocytes) and the *platelets*. These make up only a tiny volume of the blood; all the body's circulating white cells would not even fill a bartender's jigger, and all its platelets could easily fit into a teaspoon. In contrast, all the body's red cells would overflow a half-gallon milk carton. Leukocytes are involved in the immune response to foreign substances, and platelets are necessary for proper clotting of the blood. While these cells are not directly germane to our discussion of anemia, they will be discussed briefly in later chapters.

HEMOGLOBIN

The only function of the red blood cell is to keep *hemoglobin* healthy and happy. With no DNA-containing nucleus, the erythrocyte cannot reproduce itself or program itself to adapt to various challenges by synthesizing new proteins. With no mitochondria (tiny sacs in the cytoplasm filled with sugar-burning enzymes) it cannot generate the large amount of energy enjoyed by almost all other cells of the body. By allowing for the relatively limited role it performs in physiology, the red cell has its work cut out for it in caring for hemoglobin, a most fastidious customer. Hemoglobin is a protein that serves as a carrier for oxygen from the lungs to the tissues. To work properly, the hemoglobin has to hold on to oxygen molecules with just the right amount of force. If the hemoglobin molecule binds the oxygen molecules too loosely, then it will not be capable of picking them up at the lungs. If it binds the oxygen too tightly, then when it gets out to the tissues it will not release the oxygen to the tissues that need it. To perform such a delicate balancing act, the hemoglobin molecule takes advantage of its unusual physical structure (fig. 1.1). Each hemoglobin molecule consists of 4 smaller protein molecules, called *globin subunits*. There are 2 alpha and 2 beta subunits in each molecule. Each subunit partially encloses an unusual molecule called *heme*. Heme is similar to a class of compounds called *porphyrins*, which are widely found in nature in various roles. Chlorophyll, the light-capturing component of green plants, is an example of a porphyrin-based molecule. One peculiar property of porphyrins is their willingness to bind atoms of heavy metals. In the case of heme, that heavy metal is iron. Each heme molecule (4 per hemoglobin molecule) contains 1 atom of iron. Although 4 atoms of iron may seem a trivial amount in an enormous protein molecule (the protein part of hemoglobin weighs almost 300 times more than the iron it contains), iron is an absolutely essential component of hemoglobin. Without iron, there is no hemoglobin. Since without hemoglobin there is no blood, iron is an essential component of vertebrate life. (Iron will be discussed in detail in chapter 3.)

When an oxygen molecule binds to a hemoglobin molecule, the latter changes shape very slightly, which causes the next

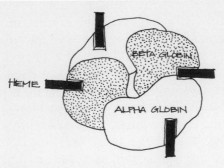

FIG. 1.1. The structure of the hemoglobin molecule

oxygen molecule to bind to the hemoglobin molecule even more avidly. This again causes a change in shape and again increases the willingness of the hemoglobin molecule to bind with oxygen. The process continues until the hemoglobin molecule has bound a total of 4 oxygen molecules, at which time the hemoglobin is full; it can bind no more oxygen. When the oxygen-laden hemoglobin gets out to the tissues of the body, it begins to drop off its oxygen load. The first oxygen molecule is given up reluctantly, but each subsequent one is released more easily than the last. What is the physiological advantage of this phenomenon?

The answer lies in a basic observation, well known to chemists and physicists, called the law of mass action. Essentially, this law states that chemical substances move spontaneously from areas of greater concentration to areas of lesser concentration. In the lungs, oxygen moves from its high concentration in the inhaled air toward the red blood cells, which have a low concentration. The problem is that, as oxygen moves into the red cells, its concentration becomes greater in the blood, and, because of the law of mass action, it is progressively more difficult to get oxygen to move from the lung to the blood. Accordingly, evolution has provided all vertebrates with the gift of hemoglobin. As the hemoglobin picks up oxygen from the lungs and gets more saturated, the changes in the hemoglobin molecule's shape force it to chemically bind oxygen more tightly, so that, despite the law of mass action, oxygen continues rapidly crossing over into the blood.

Out in the peripheral tissues, the reverse situation takes place. With the high concentration of oxygen in the blood initially assuring transfer of oxygen from blood to tissues, the law of mass action tries to slow this transfer down as the concentration of oxygen in the blood decreases. Once again hemoglobin saves the day, as it increasingly unbinds and delivers oxygen molecules with each of the oxygens that is stripped from it.

So it is clear that hemoglobin has to have its peculiar structure for proper oxygen transport, even if that structure turns out to be very delicate. Just as schoolyard bullies like to pick on the weakest classmate, almost any type of natural or artificial toxic substance can cause the hemoglobin molecule to denature (be permanently altered so that it does not work). The task of the red cell is to protect hemoglobin from these assailants. It has to continually synthesize certain molecules that destroy the toxins, and also has to maintain the correct pH (the degree of acidity or alkalinity of a liquid). It even has to keep the iron atoms happy. If an iron atom loses even one electron (which it likes to do if left to its own delinquent devices), the hemoglobin in which it resides turns into something called methemoglobin, which is totally worthless as an oxygen carrier.

HOW THE BODY ADAPTS TO ANEMIA

The various causes of different types of anemia will be discussed in later chapters, but first it is important to consider what all anemias and people with anemia have in common. As stated earlier, *anemia is the condition characterized by an abnormal decrease in the body's total red blood cell mass.* There are two possibilities as to what happens then to the blood's physical properties. The first is that, as the mass of red cells goes down, so does the total volume of blood. In fact, this is exactly what happens whenever there is heavy bleeding over a short period of time, whether from a wound or a disease (such as a bleeding ulcer). When this happens, the blood is just as thick and concentrated as it is in the normal state, but there is less of it left in the body. This is referred to as *anemia of acute blood loss.* While this does strictly fit our definition of anemia, it is in something of a category of its own, mostly because the loss in red cell mass plays second fiddle to the loss of total blood volume. When acute bleeding occurs, the most important thing for doctors to do is to maintain blood volume, even if they have to use fluids other than blood. This does not replace the lost red cell mass, to be sure, but it does keep the patient from going into shock, which can be irreversible. This is why the first thing that is done for severely injured patients, such as at the scene of an accident, is to get an IV going. The IV (intravenous) fluids can replenish the circulating fluid volume long enough for the patient to get to a hospital, where a blood transfusion can be given.

The second possibility surrounding the loss of total red cell mass is the one that is typically associated with all anemias except anemia of acute blood loss. In this scenario, the loss of red cells is gradual over weeks or months, so that the body has time to adapt to it. In this case, the body starts its own "IV" and adds water to the circulating blood volume. It does this by causing the kidneys to hold on to the water that is taken in by normal drinking. As more water is added to the plasma, and as the mass of red cells continues to decrease, the blood becomes thinner, i. e., less syrupy and more watery. To a point this is a favorable adaptation. Because thinner blood can travel through the tiny capillaries faster than thick blood, in the early stages of anemia the blood actually becomes more efficient at delivering oxygen to the tissues. However, as with many quick fixes the body employs to deal with problems, things eventually go awry. As the blood continues to thin out, less and less oxygen-laden hemoglobin is presented to the tissues per unit time. The result is oxygen starvation at the cellular level. But the body, not ready to give up yet, has several tricks up its sleeve:

(1) *Increased cardiac output.* The volume of blood the heart pumps through itself per unit time is called the cardiac output. In the normal resting state, the heart pumps about 5 liters of blood every minute, abbreviated 5 L/min. This means that the heart is easily capable of pumping the body's total blood volume through its chambers in one minute. Actually it is capable of much more than that. When there is a greater demand for oxygen, as during vigorous exercise, the heart can increase its output manyfold, to as much as 30 L/min. It does this by increasing not only the number of beats per minute (the heart

rate) but also the volume of blood pumped with each stroke (the stroke volume). Mathematically, the cardiac output can be calculated by multiplying the heart rate times the stroke volume. In anemia, the cardiac output increases, and that allows more hemoglobin to be exposed to the peripheral tissues, making up for the decreased hemoglobin concentration. Accordingly, the heart rate increases, which gives us one of the cardinal clinical manifestations of anemia, *tachycardia*, or fast heart rate.

The heart does not act alone to increase the cardiac output. It has to have cooperation from the peripheral tissues and the blood itself. If nothing changes in the body but the heart rate and stroke volume, the heart will be trying to pump blood faster into a fixed, unchanging bed of blood vessels. This is like trying to squeeze thick dishwasher detergent gel out of its container by pushing harder. The only way to make the gel dribble out faster is to increase the pressure. Analogously, in the body, to push more blood through an ungiving vascular bed would require a higher blood pressure. Higher blood pressure would cause the heart to work harder, because it would have to pump against a high pressure head, just like a muscle has to work harder to lift a heavier weight. Clearly this is not in the best interest of the body. Fortunately, the blood pressure is kept from going up by two factors. The first is the viscosity of anemic blood. Viscosity is the quality of a fluid which tends to cause it to resist being propelled through a tube or opening. Thin, anemic blood is less viscous than normal blood and can be pushed through the vascular bed with less pressure. The second factor is the blood vessels themselves. The wall of each small artery or vein contains one or more layers of muscle capable of responding to nerve signals by contracting. This causes the vessel to close down to a smaller caliber and be more resistant to the flow of blood. Other nerve impulses cause the muscles to relax, letting the vessels expand to a wider caliber and allowing more blood to flow with less resistance. In the anemic patient, the brain sends signals to the muscles around the small vessels telling them to relax and open up. The result is less impediment to the flow of blood. Therefore, because of less peripheral vessel resistance and thinner, less viscous blood, the cardiac output can rise without causing the blood pressure to go up.

(2) *Redistribution of blood flow.* The various organs of the body are quite capable of cutting deals among themselves when times are bad. In the case of anemia, all the organs conjoin to protect the two most oxygen-demanding organs in the body, the brain and the heart. If these organs don't get enough oxygen, the rest of the body is in real trouble. Fortunately, two other organs can get by without nearly as much blood as they normally enjoy in good times. The first of these is the skin. As a response to anemia, small blood vessels in the skin contract, causing a greater resistance to the flow of blood than is present in more vital organs. Since the blood being pumped out of the heart will preferentially follow the path of least resistance, it will go through the more vital organs faster than it will through skin with contracted vessels. The result is a partial diversion of blood from the skin to other organs. The second organ which sacrifices its right to blood supply is the kidney. Now the kidney is a very vital organ, to be sure, but it is normally endowed with much more blood flow than it needs to stay alive and function properly. Both kidneys, taken together, weight about 350 grams (or about ½ of 1 percent of the total body weight), but they receive 20 percent of the cardiac output, or about 1 liter per minute. Gram for gram, then, the kidneys receive 50 times the cardiac output of the body as a whole. Clearly they could give up some of that for the benefit of their fellow organs, and as part of the adaptation to anemia, they do so.

The diversion of blood flow from the skin causes one of the cardinal clinical features of anemia—*pallor.* Pallor is the pale color observed in the skin of a light-skinned anemic individual, and in the mucous membranes and nailbeds of all anemic individuals, light-skinned or otherwise. It should be noted that anemic patients are pale not because their blood is thin (anemic blood is just as opaque and highly colored as normal blood), but because the diversion of blood means that there is less of it in the skin, and more of the pale color of bloodless human tissue shows through.

(3) *Decrease of hemoglobin-oxygen affinity.* Earlier we discussed how the affinity (or the "willingness" to bind) between oxygen and hemoglobin changed with the number of oxygen molecules gained or lost by hemoglobin. It turns out that hemoglobin-oxygen affinity can be accomplished by other chemical means as well. There is a simple organic acid, called 2,3-diphosphoglycerate (2,3-DPG) that is elaborated within the red cell under anemic conditions. This 2,3-DPG causes hemoglobin to bind oxygen less avidly and to give up as much to the starved tissues as possible. Of course, the other side of the coin is that oxygen is more difficult to pick up in the lungs, but, since the respiratory system is not the main concern in an anemic patient, something has to give, and the healthy system ends up taking up the slack for the sick one.

WHEN COMPENSATION FAILS: THE CLINICALLY ANEMIC PERSON

A recurring theme in the study of disease is the sequence of events by which the body withstands some sort of insult (in the case of anemia, the decrease of red cell mass) by engineering various physiological workarounds to compensate for the damage done. Fortunately the body's various systems have a tremendous amount of reserve function to draw on to support these schemes. The down side is that when the insult becomes so great that the healthy systems, which are stretched to their limits, cannot overcome it, then the whole physiology comes crashing down like a house of cards. The result is a sick person in need of medical attention. In anemia, such a person appears with a characteristic constellation of symptoms and signs. These are listed below, along with the physiologic phenomenon responsible for each.

(1) *Pallor* is due to the shunting of blood flow away from the skin, as discussed above.

(2) *Tachycardia*, or fast heart rate, results from the increased cardiac output, also discussed above.

(3) *Dyspnea (shortness of breath) occurs on exertion.* Although the respiratory system in the anemic person is healthy, the tissues out in the body are starved for oxygen, because there is not enough hemoglobin to get it to them. When they need even more oxygen, as in a period of strenuous exercise, they send signals to the respiratory system asking it to deliver more. The respiratory system responds by increasing the depth and rate of breathing, which the anemic person experiences as shortness of breath.

(4) *Easy fatigability* is an effect of oxygen starvation at the tissue level.

(5) *Dizziness and fainting* are due to relative lack of oxygen in the brain.

(6) *Tinnitus* means the perception of noises which do not exist, or "ringing in the ears." In the anemic patient, this may actually be more of a buzzing or roaring. One possible explanation for this is that the cardiac output is so increased that the rushing of the blood through the vessels in the region of the ear is perceived as sound. Oxygen starvation of the brain cells is an alternative explanation.

(7) *Headaches* can be a symptom of anemia, although the exact cause is unknown.

(8) *Miscellaneous symptoms* include dimmed vision (which suggests oxygen starvation of the brain), loss of appetite, nausea, and constipation.

(9) *Heart failure* may occur. The cardiac output can increase only up to a certain point. After that, if the heart is called on to deliver even more blood per minute, it fails. When this happens the heart is unable to pump through all the blood presented to it by the veins, causing a buildup in pressure there; the blood then backs up into the capillaries. In this high-pressure environment, fluid from the plasma of the blood begins to seep out of the capillaries into the tissues. When this happens in the peripheral

tissues of the body, swelling occurs, a condition referred to as edema. This swelling is seen particularly around the ankles (pedal edema) and over the lower back (sacral edema). When edema occurs in the lungs, the fluid not only causes the thin walls of the alveoli to swell, thus stiffening the lung and making inhaling more difficult, but it also fills up the alveolar sacs themselves, interfering with the exchange of oxygen and carbon dioxide. This is called pulmonary edema, and it is a dire event in the clinical course of the severely anemic patient. Without treatment (or with unskillful treatment) such a condition will quickly lead to the patient's demise.

Now that we have a person with clinically full-blown anemia in need of medical care, we will look at how doctors make a diagnosis and how they classify each person's case for proper management.

2. How Is Anemia Diagnosed?

Although clinical diagnosis is an expert skill that takes years of intensive effort to develop, the fundamental intellectual functions involved differ little from those we use when picking out a friend in a large crowd. Through pattern recognition, experienced physicians are able to make about 90 percent of their diagnoses. They ask a few questions (take a history) and make some visual, auditory, and tactile observations of the person's body (perform a physical examination). From this relatively brief encounter, the doctor establishes that a familiar pattern exists, and makes a presumptive diagnosis. Since the human body is enormously complex, however, nature can throw the doctor quite a few curves, and the presumptive diagnosis is not always right. Accordingly, the physician formulates a list of other, less likely diseases to be ruled out by various tests. This list, together with the presumptive diagnosis, is called the differential diagnosis, or just the "differential." Each test is designed to rule out one or more of the incorrect items on the differential diagnosis, so that only the correct one will be left. Most tests fall into one of two categories, clinical laboratory tests and imaging. Imaging, which includes plain X-rays, CT scans, and MRI scans, is very important to medicine in general but is of only peripheral interest in the differential diagnosis of anemia. Clinical lab tests, on the other hand, figure prominently in the diagnosis and proper categorization of the anemias.

THE CLINICAL LABORATORY

According to the popular concept, a laboratory is a room filled with complicated glassware, miles of tubing, huge computers, and eccentric, white-coated scientists. In fact, the modern clinical laboratory bears little resemblance to what is shown in science fiction movies. The familiar microscope is readily recognizable, but the rest of the hardware looks more like an assembly of featureless boxes of various sizes. These machines are highly automated and are operated through a computer interface typically consisting of a keyboard and monitor identical to those on a desktop computer workstation.

People who work in the lab are highly trained professionals. Two categories of laboratorians do most of the work. The first is the medical technologist (MT or med tech). Most MTs are graduates of four-year colleges and have baccalaureate degrees in medical technology. Their courses of study include general and analytical chemistry, general biology, microbiology, hematology, blood banking, medical microscopy, and computer applications. The MT training program is exceedingly demanding and covers basically everything first- and second-year medical students study, with the exception of pharmacology, physical diagnosis, and detailed anatomy. In addition, MTs must learn certain subjects (such as microbiology and blood banking) in considerably greater detail than their counterparts in medical school. It has been my observation that former med techs make the best medical students.

The second line-level laboratory worker is the medical laboratory technician, or MLT. These are usually graduates of two-year associate-degree training programs run by community colleges. Many MLT students are people seeking second careers (after raising families or working in unskilled jobs) and are drawn from the segment of society well educated in the "school of hard knocks." They bring with them not only an interest in and talent for the sciences, but an enthusiasm and dedication typically seen only in mature individuals who have had to work hard for everything they have achieved.

The medical specialty that deals with the clinical laboratory is clinical pathology. To become a clinical pathologist in the United States, a physician must undertake a four-year residency training program and pass a certifying examination given by the American Board of Pathology. Clinical pathologists do not actually run most lab tests, as their focus is on making diagnoses using laboratory techniques, assuring the quality of the lab's work, designing strategies for how tests should be run, and performing consultations at the request of primary care physicians.

Clinical laboratories are usually divided into sections based on the type of work done at each. The typical hematology section, which is the one we are interested in here, has several tools or machines with which the laboratorians work. The clinical microscope is familiar to most people. It allows blood specimens to be examined at magnifications between 100 and 1000 times life size. As mentioned earlier, blood cells have to be stained before they can be seen in detail, so a lab usually has a staining machine. The centerpiece of the typical hematology section is the automated cell counter. This is a very expensive, computer-driven machine that rapidly and accurately counts blood cells and determines their size and shape.

BASIC HEMATOLOGY LAB TESTS

The three cardinal red cell measurements

Here again is the definition of anemia given in chapter 1: it is *any condition characterized by an abnormal decrease in the body's total red blood cell mass*. Obviously, determining the mass of a patient's red cells by removing all of them from the body and weighing them would not be practical. Fortunately for us, the body's response to anemia makes the job of determining red cell mass relatively easy. Remember that the body reacts to developing anemia by adding water to the blood to maintain its volume. This results in blood that is more dilute in terms of the number of red cells per unit volume of whole blood. By measuring the level of dilution of the blood, we can indirectly measure the mass of red cells in the circulation. The most straightforward way to make this determination is to count the number of red cells in a known volume of whole blood. This test, the first cardinal red cell measurement, is called the *red blood cell count*, or just "RBC count." Normally there are between 4,700,000 and 6,100,000 red cells in a microliter of an adult male's blood. Thus, the normal range or reference range for the RBC count in a male is 4.7 to 6.1 million cells per microliter, expressed in shorthand as 4.7–6.1 million/μL (the lower-case Greek letter μ is used for "micro"). For the normal woman, the reference range is 4.2–5.4 million/μL. An anemic person would be expected to have an RBC count under the lower limit of the reference range for his or her age and sex.

The problem with using the RBC count as a test for anemia is that all red cells are not created equal. In the various types of anemia and other hematologic conditions, the size and weight of each red cell can vary markedly. According to our definition, red cell mass is the sole determinant of anemia, and simply counting red cells does not give us an indication of red cell mass. For instance, if the number of red cells is normal, but the mass of each cell is abnormally low, then the person is still anemic, despite a normal RBC count. Clearly, we need a test to measure the mass of the red cells in a unit volume of blood. Fortunately, this is not difficult because of the very simple chemical composition of the red cell. RBCs are composed almost entirely of hemoglobin; thus, as the concentration of hemoglobin in a unit of whole blood decreases, so does the red cell mass. This brings us to the second cardinal red cell measurement, the *hemoglobin concentration in whole blood*, or simply "the hemoglobin." It is very difficult to measure the concentration of hemoglobin in individual red cells, so the first step is to pop all the red cells and let the hemoglobin flow out into the blood sample, where it becomes evenly distributed in the plasma. This process is called hemolysis (from *hemo*, "blood," and *lysis*, "destruction"). Since hemoglobin is a colored substance, its concentration should be easily measured by the shining of a light through a given thickness of the specimen to determine how much light is blocked. This is the basis of an analytic technique called colorimetry. The lower the concentration of the colored substance, the more light shines through. The only problem is that, when hemoglobin is released from the red cells, it goes berserk chemically and starts to break down, losing some of its light-absorbing qualities. The way around this is to chemically transform the released hemoglobin into a much more stable, but still colored, substance called cyanmethemoglobin. The solution of cyanmethemoglobin is then analyzed by colorimetry, and, after a few mathematical calculations, the original concentration of hemoglobin in the person's blood can be determined. A normal adult man's blood contains between 14 and 18 grams of hemoglobin in 1 deciliter of whole blood (a deciliter is 1/10 of a liter). This reference range is then expressed as 14–18 g/dL. The corresponding range for an adult woman is 12–16 g/dL. A chronically anemic person has a hemoglobin less than the lower figure of the appropriate reference range. As a matter of practice, we usually use the 12 g/dL figure for both men and women for our clinical definition of anemia. We can now state a new, more practical definition for anemia that is used by most doctors: *anemia is any condition characterized by a hemoglobin of less than 12 g/dL.* Not every doctor uses this definition all the time. Some doctors allow elderly people a hemoglobin slightly lower than 12 g/dL without initiating a diagnostic workup, while others stick to the stated normal range for every adult, regardless of age. Another source of variation is the clinical laboratory, since not all labs have exactly the same reference ranges.

The hemoglobin is one of the most accurate and reproducible of all laboratory tests. Because of this, it is used as the primary test for diagnosing and following the course of anemia. It can also be used to classify the severity of anemia. A hemoglobin between 10 and 12 g/dL is *mild anemia*; between 7 and 10 g/dL, *moderate anemia*; and less than 7 g/dL, *severe anemia*. Mild anemia usually causes no symptoms and is picked up by lab testing only. Moderate anemia may produce symptoms with exertion or other stress. Severe anemia may produce symptoms at rest.

There is a third cardinal red cell measurement that is useful in the classification of anemias, the *hematocrit*. Another, more illuminating, name for hematocrit is *packed cell volume*, or PCV. This is defined as the fraction of the volume of whole blood occupied by the red blood cells. Hematocrit is therefore a measurement of volume, not mass. For example, if 100 milliliters of a person's blood contains 25 milliliters of red cells, then the hematocrit is $^{25}/_{100}$, or 25 percent. This figure can also be expressed as a unitless fraction, 0.25, or as a volume unit, 0.25 L/L (liters red cells per liter whole blood). The old-fashioned way of determining the hematocrit is to draw up a small amount of the person's blood into a narrow glass tube and spin the tube in a centrifuge. The centrifugal force, which is many times that of gravity, causes all of the red cells, which are denser than the plasma, to pack down into the bottom of the tube, leaving a clear column of plasma on top. The length of the column of red cells is divided by the length of the column of the whole specimen to give the hematocrit. Modern automated techniques for measuring hematocrit actually determine the exact volume of each of thousands of red cells in a specimen of known volume, add up those volumes, and divide that sum by the total volume of the specimen to get the result.

The hematocrit was a more prominent diagnostic tool in the days when medical students and residents had to do much of the admission lab work on their patients. Performing this test by the traditional centrifugation method does not require a lot of delicate hardware, or even much manual skill. Accordingly, it was especially suited to dingy, poorly maintained student labs in the large charity hospitals where so many of us had our professional beginnings. Back then, the hematocrit was the major test used to diagnose and follow the course of anemia. Nowadays, with automated labs and better laboratory services, the hemoglobin has taken its place. We still routinely perform hematocrits when anemia is suspected, because it provides data useful in the calculation of red cell indices, described below.

The red cell indices

At first, it might seem that the three cardinal red cell measurements are redundant. After all, in most anemic people, all three measurements—RBC count, hemoglobin, and hematocrit—are abnormally low. As anemia gets worse, they all fall, and as the anemia responds to proper treatment, they all come back up. It turns out that, while all three tests tend to run in parallel, those "parallel" lines are not always perfectly straight. In one type of anemia, for example, the red cell count, while low, is even lower than would be expected for the observed level of hemoglobin. This is because in that particular type of anemia (called macrocytic anemia), the red cells, while decreased in number, are abnormally large in volume. The low red cell count, therefore, is partially compensated for by the larger volume of the cell, giving a higher-than-expected hemoglobin. Thus, it is very important to classify anemias based in part on the size of the red cells and the hemoglobin content thereof. To facilitate this classification, a set of three calculated *red cell indices* has been devised.

The first of the red cell indices is the *mean corpuscular volume* (MCV), which is the average volume of a given person's red cells. The MCV is numerically calculated by dividing the hematocrit by the RBC count and multiplying by a unit conversion factor. The reference range for MCV is 80 to 94 femtoliters (a femtoliter is one quadrillionth of a liter), or, as commonly abbreviated, 80–94 fL. An anemia in which the MCV is below this range is a *microcytic* anemia. One in which the MCV falls within the reference range is a *normocytic* anemia, while an anemia with an MCV higher than the reference range is a *macrocytic* anemia. Any given case of anemia, then, can be classified as microcytic, normocytic, or macrocytic, based on the MCV. This is an important classification, as it serves to narrow down considerably the differential diagnosis of anemia.

The second of the red cell indices is the *mean corpuscular hemoglobin* (MCH), which is the average mass of hemoglobin in each of the person's red cells. The MCH is calculated by dividing the hemoglobin concentration of whole blood by the RBC count and multiplying by a unit conversion factor. The reference range for MCH is 27 to 31 picograms (a picogram is one trillionth of a gram), abbreviated 27–31 pg. It turns out that the MCH is not a very important red cell index, because it tends to parallel the MCV. This is to be expected, since a small red cell contains less hemoglobin than a large one. This will be the last mention of the MCH.

The third red cell index is the *mean corpuscular hemoglobin concentration* (MCHC), which is the average concentration of hemoglobin in a person's red cells. It is calculated by dividing the whole blood hemoglobin concentration by the hematocrit and applying a unit conversion factor. The reference range is 32 to 36 grams per deciliter, abbreviated 32–36 g/dL. Anemia in which the MCHC is lower than that range is a *hypochromic* anemia; that with MCHC within the reference range is a *normochromic* anemia; and an anemia with a high MCHC is a *hyperchromic* anemia. Hyperchromic anemias are very rare and will not be considered further. The two important classifications of anemia based on the MCHC, then, are hypochromic and normochromic anemias.

CYTOMETRIC CLASSIFICATION OF ANEMIA

After the diagnosis of anemia is made (by determining that the person has a low hemoglobin), the next challenge for the physician is to determine what type of anemia it is. Using the red cell indices, a given case can be classified into one of three broad categories, based on the average size and hemoglobin content of the red cells, as measured by the MCV and MCHC, respectively. This is called the *cytometric classification of anemia* ("cytometric" means "cell size"). The three categories are:

(1) *Microcytic, hypochromic anemia.* The MCV and MCHC are both low, indicating that the red cells are small and pale (i.e., have a lowered concentration of hemoglobin). The major types of anemia that fall into this category are iron deficiency (chapter 3) and thalassemia (chapter 6).

(2) *Macrocytic, normochromic anemia.* The MCV is high, but the MCHC is normal, indicating that the cells are larger than normal but have normal hemoglobin concentration. The major types of anemia in this category are anemias of folate and vitamin B_{12} deficiency (chapter 4) and refractory anemia (chapter 7).

(3) *Normocytic, normochromic anemia.* The MCV and MCHC are both normal, which means that the cells are of normal size and possess a normal concentration of hemoglobin. Unfortunately, this includes a very broad spectrum of anemias, some of which are discussed in chapters 5, 6, and 7.

IN SUMMARY

From a practical standpoint, the diagnosis of anemia is made by use of lab tests that determine the three cardinal red cell measurements—RBC count, hemoglobin, and hematocrit—with the hemoglobin being the most important and most reliable. Those measurements allow calculations to be made that yield the three red cell indices—MCV, MCH, and MCHC, with the MCH being relatively unimportant. From those indices, the anemia is placed into one of three cytometric classifications—microcytic, hypochromic; macrocytic, normochromic; and normocytic, normochromic.

Once the cytometric classification is made, the doctor must continue to narrow down the differential diagnosis until the nature of the anemia can be exactly determined. This often involves additional laboratory tests. We will deal with some of these tests throughout the remainder of this book, as we consider each of the major types of anemias.

3. Iron Deficiency Anemia

Briefly stated, iron deficiency anemia (IDA) is *that anemia caused by an inadequate supply of iron available to the bone marrow*, where red cells are made. As we shall see, this can be due to (1) failure to take in enough iron or (2) accelerated loss of iron from the body. Under the cytometric classification of anemia given in the previous chapter, IDA is a *microcytic, hypochromic anemia*. Before getting into the pathogenesis (origin and development) of IDA, we shall consider the role of iron in metabolism.

THE CHEMICAL COMPOSITION OF THE BODY

The human body is an enormously complex metabolic factory that is composed of thousands of different chemical compounds, which consist of chemical elements. There are 92 naturally occurring elements, and, of those, only a fraction are involved in human physiology. The vast majority of the body's compounds consist predominantly of some combination of the elements carbon, hydrogen, oxygen, nitrogen, sulfur, and phosphorus. In addition, potassium, sodium, chlorine, calcium, and magnesium play important roles in regulation of fluid balance and maintenance of excitable tissues, such as nerve and muscle. All of these are "light" elements, in that they are composed of atoms with nuclei that contain few protons and neutrons. The heaviest of these, chlorine, is 17th from the bottom when the 92 elements are ranked by weight. Hydrogen, which is by far the most plentiful of the body's elements in terms of numbers of atoms, is the lightest of the 92 elements. It can be said, therefore, that the human body (and the bodies of most organisms, in fact) is composed almost entirely of light elements.

However, the heavier elements have not been totally shunned in the vagaries of biological evolution. Iodine is the heaviest element in human metabolism (ranking 26th from the top of the 92 elements) and is essential for the proper function of the thyroid gland. A small number of other heavy elements have found their way into living systems as substances which are absolutely necessary for normal function, but only in very small amounts. These are called trace elements. Since most of the heavy elements in biological organisms are physically metallic (the exception being iodine), they are often referred to as trace metals. The most important trace metals in humans are given in the table below, with the typical quantity of each in a 70-kilogram (154-pound) person.

Trace Metal	Amount (grams)
iron	4.0
zinc	3.0
cobalt	1.1
copper	0.25
molybdenum	0.07
manganese	0.02
chromium	0.0006
selenium	(no reliable data available)

These are, indeed, very small amounts. For instance, the 0.25 grams of copper in the average body would, if extracted and converted into its pure metallic form, make up a spherical bead measuring only about 4 millimeters (⅙ inch) in diameter. The body contains such a scant amount of chromium that all of the chromium in the entire human species (world population 5.9 billion) would constitute a cube of purified metal no more than 79 centimeters (31 inches) on a side. All of the trace metals, including iron, share two important physiological properties: (1) each is absolutely essential for normal health, and (2) each is toxic if present in excess amounts.

IRON

The most abundant of all the body's trace elements is iron; the 4 grams contained in the typical adult are equivalent to a pure metal ball measuring 1 centimeter (about 3/8 inch) in diameter. Iron does not exist in the body as a pure metal, however. It is combined with a variety of organic chemicals to form compounds that deal mostly with the storage and transport of oxygen. One of those compounds is hemoglobin. As mentioned in chapter 1, each hemoglobin molecule contains 4 molecules of heme, each of which contains 1 atom of iron. Although iron is a much heavier element than all the others that make up hemoglobin (carbon, hydrogen, oxygen, nitrogen, and sulfur), it is so overwhelmed by the sheer number of other atoms that it makes up only about 1/3 of 1 percent of the mass of hemoglobin. It is tempting to think that a substance present in such an insignificant amount could easily be done without. In fact, hemoglobin without iron does not and cannot even exist. Iron is so important in maintaining the unstable affinity between hemoglobin and oxygen that the absence of even 1 of the 4 iron atoms of a hemoglobin molecule would make that molecule totally worthless as an oxygen carrier. The bottom line is that iron is absolutely required for the synthesis of hemoglobin, and, since red cells are little more than bags of hemoglobin, iron is absolutely required for the production of red cells.

About 2/3 of the body's iron resides in hemoglobin. About 1/7 is held in storage, mostly in the marrow, from which developing red cells can draw as their hemoglobin content is synthesized. The remainder of the iron is used mostly in myoglobin, a hemoglobin-like substance in muscle capable of storing oxygen temporarily. Trace amounts of the body's iron are found throughout many tissues, where it participates in a variety of chemical reactions involving oxygen.

A QUICK TOUR OF THE DIGESTIVE SYSTEM

As mentioned earlier, iron deficiency anemia is caused either by insufficient iron taken in or by the loss of it at such a rate that it cannot be replaced. The only way the body can acquire iron is through the diet, and the only significant way the body normally gets rid of excess iron is by excreting it in the feces. In cases of IDA caused by accelerated loss of iron, the condition is often (but not always) due to diseases of the alimentary tract, from which blood seeps and escapes into the feces, taking iron along with it. In any case, the story of IDA is closely linked with the story of the digestive system, so a brief description of that system is appropriate here.

The digestive system consists of the alimentary tract (synonyms: gastrointestinal or digestive tract, GI tract, gut) and the glandular organs that secrete into it. These glandular organs are the salivary glands, liver and pancreas. The GI tract itself consists of the mouth, esophagus, stomach, duodenum, small bowel, colon (large bowel), and rectum (fig. 3.1). The mouth kicks off the digestive process by crushing and shearing the food into smaller pieces (chewing) and lubricating it with mucus to prepare it for the esophagus. The salivary glands also contribute here by secreting an enzyme, amylase, which starts the job of breaking down carbohydrate molecules in food. The function of the esophagus is simply to convey food from the mouth to the stomach and keep it from coming back up. The esophagus is a classic example of the organ you never much appreciate until it goes haywire. The stomach continues the digestive process by pouring out large amounts of acid, as well as an enzyme, pepsin, that breaks down protein.

The contents of the stomach are then expelled into the duodenum (technically the first segment of the small bowel), where digestion really gets going. Here the food is met by powerful enzymes secreted by the pancreas: trypsin, chymotrypsin, and carboxypeptidases A and B, which digest

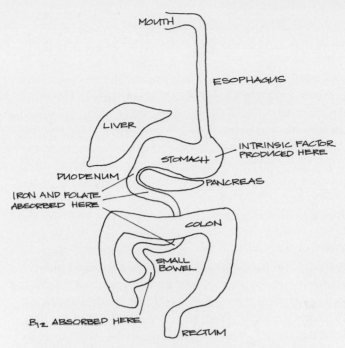

FIG. 3.1. The digestive system. Folate, B$_{12}$, and intrinsic factor are
discussed in chapter 4.

protein; amylase, which digests carbohydrates; and lipase, which
digests fat. Another important contribution to digestion is
secreted into the duodenum by the liver. This is bile, which
is a green detergent-like substance necessary to break fat into
droplets small enough for pancreatic lipase to work on it. By the
time the duodenum and its secretions get through with dinner, it
is reduced to an unrecognizable greenish-yellow goop referred
to as chyme, the nutrients of which are easily absorbed by the
internal lining (mucosa) of the small bowel with the help of yet
more digestive enzymes affixed to the mucosal surface. This
process of absorption actually begins in the duodenum and is
mostly complete by the time the chyme gets through the first
half of the small bowel, called the jejunum. The second half

of the small bowel, the ileum, is also capable of absorption, and the farthest end of the ileum (terminal ileum) is special to hematology in that this is the only place in the whole gut where vitamin B_{12} can be absorbed (see chapter 4). The colon and rectum are not capable of absorbing nutrients. The only functions they serve are to absorb water (thus conserving it) and to lubricate with mucus the now-solid feces for its final passage out of the body.

IRON INTAKE—NORMAL AND ABNORMAL

Iron is widely available in the foodstuffs consumed in modern industrialized countries. The classic foods considered high in iron are meats and dark green vegetables, but so many processed, packaged foods are fortified with extra iron that this nutrient often turns up unexpectedly, even in foods generally considered little more than empty calories. The typical daily dietary intake of iron for American adults is about 10 milligrams, which is usually more than adequate, since we need to absorb only about 1 milligram of that to keep from becoming iron deficient. The following table gives some idea as to how widely iron is distributed in what we eat.

Food Item (amount)	Iron Content (milligrams)
Corn Chex cereal (1 cup)	8.3
Kellogg's Frosted Flakes (1 cup)	6.2
liver, beef, fried (3 ounces)	5.3
Kellogg's Raisin Bran (1 cup)	5.0
black beans, cooked (1 cup)	3.6
chitterlings, pork, simmered (3 ounces)	3.1
ground beef, extra lean, cooked (3 ounces)	2.0
spaghetti, cooked, enriched (1 cup)	2.0
kale, cooked (1 cup)	1.2
Ralston Purina Sugar Frosted Flakes (1 cup)	1.0

white bread, commercial (1 large slice)   0.9
spinach, raw (1 cup)   0.8
frankfurter, beef and pork (1)   0.5
carrot (1 medium)   0.3
milk, whole (1 cup)   0.1

Obviously, it is impossible to give the iron content of the entire panoply of the foods we eat, but three messages should be clear from the table above:

(1) Iron is just about everywhere. If you eat anything vaguely resembling a balanced diet, you should be able to take in enough iron to meet a healthy body's needs. As a general rule, Western diets contain about 6 milligrams of iron per 1000 Calories.

(2) It is hard to predict how much iron various processed foods have. For instance, while Kellogg's Frosted Flakes, Ralston Purina Sugar Frosted Flakes, and Corn Chex would all seem at first glance to be nothing more than variously shaped permutations of corn meal, sugar, and salt, there is wide variation in iron content among these cereals. To know what you are getting, you have to read the label.

(3) Milk is such a poor source of iron that it would take about 5 gallons of whole milk per day to meet the 10-milligram iron allowance. Although this would certainly make the dairy industry very happy, that much milk would bring with it over 12,000 Calories (more than 5 times what a healthy adult needs, causing a weight gain of about 3 pounds per day), as well as 670 grams of fat (equivalent to about 30 slices of raw bacon).

The exact site of iron absorption is the segment of upper small intestine that includes the duodenum and the upper jejunum. Although the body usually absorbs only 1 milligram of the 10-milligram average daily intake, in states of iron deficiency the healthy digestive system is able to absorb a higher proportion to meet the challenge. The stomach does not absorb iron directly but facilitates its absorption by the secretion of gastric acid. Dietary iron is present in two forms, depending on how many electrons have been stripped from the outer shell of its atoms. An acidic environment fosters the conversion of iron from its ferric form, which cannot be absorbed, to the ferrous form, which can. If the ferric iron cannot be converted to the ferrous form by exposure to acid, then sufficient iron may not be absorbed. A common scenario is the postgastrectomy state, in which some or all of the stomach has been surgically removed. The production of normal gastric acid is impaired, and iron is poorly absorbed as a result.

A diseased duodenum or jejunum may also result in a body's failure to absorb iron because of destruction of the normal absorptive cells in the gut mucosa. This is called *malabsorption*. One of the several diseases that can cause malabsorption is gluten-sensitive enteropathy (GSE), also called celiac sprue. In GSE, the person suffers from an allergy-like hypersensitivity to a protein (gluten) found in wheat flour and some other grain products. The body's reaction to eating wheat products is to destroy cells of the mucosa of the small bowel. The result is that iron and other nutrients are not absorbed. Classic cases of GSE are characterized by a variety of nutritional problems and severe symptoms that go far beyond iron deficiency anemia. Physicians have only recently become aware that there are many more mild cases of GSE than had been thought, and these may be difficult to diagnose because of their more subtle clinical findings. Since some mild cases do not produce any findings other than IDA, doctors have to keep such a possibility in mind when presented with persons suffering from iron deficiency.

The only other way a person may fail to take in enough iron for normal red cell production is not to eat enough foods with sufficient iron content. This is very rare in the industrialized world, and only one clinical scenario of this type is encountered with any frequency—the "milk baby." As mentioned above, milk of any type, including breast milk, is a very poor iron source. Babies kept on the breast or on bottled milk for prolonged lengths of time require some type of iron supplementation. Most commercial infant formulas also contain variable amounts of added iron. Premature infants and infants born to women who themselves were iron deficient during pregnancy are especially at risk for slipping behind in iron balance during the first year of life.

IRON LOSS—NORMAL AND ABNORMAL

A general theme in physiology is "what goes in must come out," and this certainly applies to iron. Except in menstruating women, the only route by which iron is normally lost is through the feces. Since most of us absorb about 1 milligram of iron per day, then it is to be expected that 1 milligram is lost. If the amount lost is too great, over time iron deficiency anemia develops.

Menstruating women present a special problem in iron balance. The average woman of reproductive age loses about 40 milliliters of blood during each month's menstrual period. This quantity of blood contains about 16 milligrams of iron. Spread out over the typical 28-day menstrual cycle, such a loss would require an additional daily iron intake of 0.6 milligrams (16 divided by 28) to make up the deficit. This is just a drop in the bucket compared to the 10 milligrams of iron typically found in our diets, and enhanced absorption of that normally wasted iron should easily make up the difference. The problem is that not all women are average, and the amount of blood lost varies widely. Some women can lose as much as 500 milliliters (more than 1 pint) of blood per period yet still not consider themselves to be abnormal. This is a lot of blood, equivalent to 200 milligrams of iron, or 5 percent of all the body's iron. Spread out over the 28-day cycle, this amounts to an additional iron need of 7 milligrams per day. For this reason, while the U.S. Recommended Daily Allowance (USRDA) of iron for males and postmenopausal women is 10 milligrams, the USRDA for women of reproductive age is 18 milligrams. Even with a reasonable diet, and with the iron absorption mechanism ramped up into high gear, keeping up with the prodigious amount of iron loss in a heavily menstruating woman is difficult. Thus, iron deficiency anemia is the most common type of anemia in women of reproductive age. In fact, IDA is so common in this group that some physicians do not even bother to perform a complete diagnostic workup when such a woman has symptoms of anemia; they just give an iron supplement and wait to see if the anemia resolves. If there is no response to iron therapy, then a more thorough workup is undertaken.

Accelerated iron loss in men and postmenopausal women is another story altogether. In these groups, there is no way to lose significant amounts of iron except through a disease process that disrupts the integrity of the body sufficiently for blood (and its iron) to slowly leak out. In the vast majority of cases, these diseases are conditions that affect the digestive tract mucosa. Since a variety of such conditions exists, ranging in seriousness from mild inflammation to life-threatening cancer, whenever a man or postmenopausal woman appears with iron deficiency anemia, it is absolutely necessary for the doctor not only to replace the depleted iron, but also to look for the underlying cause of the iron loss. A sampling of diseases that can lead to iron deficiency follows.

(1) *Esophagitis* is inflammation of the mucosa of the esophagus. The most common cause is failure of the muscular valve between the esophagus and stomach to keep the highly acidic gastric contents from going back up, or refluxing, into the esophagus. The esophageal lining is not adapted to withstand that much acid, and inflammation, called reflux esophagitis, results. Blood slowly leaks out of the raw, inflamed areas, and iron deficiency results.

(2) *Gastritis* is inflammation of the mucosa of the stomach. There are two major causes of gastritis: one is infection with a fairly recently discovered bacterium called *Helicobacter pylori*, and the other is use of various oral medications, most notably aspirin and the class of drugs called nonsteroidal anti-inflammatory drugs (NSAIDs). There are several NSAIDs,

three of which are sold over the counter: ibuprofen (sold as Motrin, Advil, Nuprin, and Midol IB), naproxen (Aleve), and ketoprofen (Orudis KT, Actron). All of these drugs are excellent for alleviating mild pain and inflammation, but their side effects are quite real. NSAID-induced gastritis is so common that I refer to these pills, with intended dark humor, as "the gastroenterologist's little helpers."

(3) *Peptic ulcer* is a localized area of inflammation in the lining of the duodenum or stomach. The inflammation is so intense that the mucosa and underlying tissues actually break down, and a crater results. Up until the last decade, the underlying cause of peptic ulcer was unknown, but more recent investigations have pointed the finger of blame firmly at the bacterium *Helicobacter pylori.*

(4) *Benign tumors* are fairly common in the lining of the gut. The most common benign tumors of the stomach are hyperplastic polyps. These have no important medical ramifications, except that occasionally they become ulcerated, allow blood to seep out, and cause iron deficiency. The common benign tumors of the colon and rectum are the adenomas. There are two types, the tubular adenoma (also called adenomatous polyp) and the villous adenoma. Aside from bleeding chronically and causing IDA, adenomas are important in that they have the potential of turning into frank cancers if left alone (the villous adenoma having the greater risk of the two). Moreover, persons found to have an adenoma are at risk for acquiring more, with each one signaling an increased likelihood of cancer developing. Accordingly, any patient who has ever had a colonic or rectal adenoma must be followed indefinitely and monitored for recurrences.

(5) *Cancer* is the most serious cause of chronic iron loss. In the United States and Canada, the most common cancer of the GI tract is adenocarcinoma of the colon and rectum. These cancers are generally thought to be slow-growing. They begin in the mucosa and slowly eat through the wall of the gut. They can also seed off (metastasize) and cause daughter tumors in the lymph

nodes draining the GI tract, as well as in the liver. The good news is that if colorectal adenocarcinoma is surgically removed before it gets completely through the wall of the gut, the chances of cure are excellent. The second most important cancer of the gut is adenocarcinoma of the stomach. This tumor is seen more commonly in Asia and developing countries than here, but it is a more serious cancer with a relatively poor prognosis.

CLINICAL PRESENTATION OF IRON DEFICIENCY ANEMIA

A person with classic with IDA will show some combination of the symptoms and signs of anemia already discussed in chapter 1. The anemia is confirmed by basic lab tests, discussed in chapter 2. Those same basic tests will also disclose that the anemia falls into the cytometric category of *microcytic, hypochromic*, meaning that the red cells in the blood are small and lack hemoglobin. This is not surprising, as the basic molecular defect in IDA is the inability to synthesize hemoglobin. The bone marrow does its best to turn out as many red cells as it can, but those it does turn out are stunted due to lack of raw materials.

Since iron is an important participant in a variety of other chemical reactions in the body, a deficiency can lead to an assortment of clinical signs and symptoms, some of which are rather bizarre, and all of which are currently unexplainable at the molecular level:

(1) *Developmental and behavioral disorders in children* are observed in IDA. These include social withdrawal, emotional irritability, short attention span, and low scores on tests of intellectual function. Adults also probably experience dysfunctions of this type, but people in that age group are more difficult to assess.

(2) *Pica* is the compulsive chewing or eating of objects or substances other than food. Some of the varieties of pica are so common that they are described by specific medical terms. The

abnormal eating of clay, ice, and starch is called, respectively, geophagia, pagophagia, and amylophagia. Other objects of the pica victim's craving may include paper, cardboard, burnt match heads, and toothpaste. A person may be embarrassed to talk about pica, so it is important for the doctor to attempt to draw out this diagnostically important information.

(3) *Koilonychia* is a relatively uncommon manifestation of IDA in which the nails develop an abnormal curvature. In the fully developed case, the fingernails, when viewed from the back of the hand, look like the inside surfaces of spoons. The nails are also brittle and cracked.

(4) *Glossal atrophy* is a condition in which the lining of the tongue becomes thin and wasted. The normal velvety surface of the tongue is replaced by a thin, smooth, shiny surface that lets the color of blood show through. The appearance of the tongue is described as "red and beefy." The thinned lining is also more liable to be traumatized, resulting in painful fissures.

(5) *Esophageal webs* are shelves of tissue that form in the esophagus and interfere with swallowing. These webs are easily irritated, and the chronic irritation can lead to cancer of the esophagus in a minority of cases.

LABORATORY CONFIRMATION OF IDA

There are several microcytic, hypochromic anemias besides IDA. Accordingly, it is important for a physician to rule out those others before making the definitive diagnosis. The most direct way to do this is to establish that the patient's total body iron stores are depleted. If not, then there is still iron in storage that could be used to make red cells, so the anemia must be due to some other cause. Since iron is stored in the marrow, the most direct way to check is to remove some marrow and examine it under the microscope, in what is called a bone marrow aspiration and biopsy (see appendix D for a full description). However, the expense, inconvenience, and pain of this procedure make it impractical for the simple measuring of iron stores, except in the most complicated and confusing of cases. Fortunately there are cheaper and less painful ways of determining whether iron stores are depleted, the most straightforward being the serum iron level, a routine, inexpensive lab test. As the body becomes more deficient in iron, the serum iron level falls.

Iron is present in the serum (the liquid part of the blood remaining after all cells and clotting proteins have been removed) bound to a special transport protein called *transferrin*. As the body becomes deficient in iron, the liver produces more transferrin, as if attempting to transport whatever iron can be absorbed from the gut to the marrow, where it can be incorporated into red cells. The result is an increased amount of transferrin in the serum. We can measure transferrin in the clinical laboratory, either directly or indirectly, by measuring the amount of iron that can be bound by serum proteins. This latter test is called total iron binding capacity, or TIBC. Whichever measurement technique is used, transferrin and TIBC represent the same thing, and both are expected to become elevated in iron deficiency. As the serum iron level decreases, and TIBC/transferrin increase, the ratio of iron to transferrin decreases. This calculated value is called the percent saturation of iron. Normally, this figure is about 30 percent, but in most well-established cases of IDA, it falls below 10 percent.

Serum iron and transferrin levels are useful, but their diagnostic value can be thrown off by various coexistent disease states. Fortunately, there is yet another test for depleted iron stores, the ferritin level. Ferritin is the main protein in the body that binds iron for storage. The more iron there is in storage, the more ferritin exists to bind it. A minute amount of ferritin leaks out of storage and floats around in the serum, where it can be measured in the clinical lab. As storage iron decreases, then, the serum ferritin level decreases. Again, ferritin is not a foolproof diagnostic tool, as certain disease states can raise ferritin levels into the normal or high range even in the face of iron deficiency.

Nevertheless, given the acumen of an experienced physician, the cooperation of a communicative patient, and the appropriate use of the clinical laboratory, most cases of iron deficiency anemia can be accurately diagnosed rapidly and inexpensively.

The results of standard lab tests in a typical case of iron deficiency anemia are summarized in the following table:

Test	Expected Result
hemoglobin	low
MCV	low (microcytic)
MCHC	low (hypochromic)
serum iron	low
serum transferrin (or TIBC)	high
percent iron saturation	low
serum ferritin	low

TREATMENT OF IDA

Fortunately, iron deficiency responds vigorously to treatment, and the treatment itself is easy and inexpensive. Most cases can be treated with a simple iron-containing oral drug called ferrous sulfate. Although the pharmaceutical industry has come up with myriad iron preparations, all of which are more expensive than ferrous sulfate, these are usually not necessary. Some people complain of stomach pains and indigestion from ferrous sulfate pills, but these symptoms can usually be avoided if the daily dose is taken in divided amounts during meals. The expected response to iron therapy is a rise in blood hemoglobin by an increment of at least 2 grams per deciliter within 3 to 4 weeks. If the patient fails to respond, then all the clinical data should be reevaluated in an effort to find out if there is some other problem causing the anemia. Many cases of thalassemia minor (see chapter 6) have been misdiagnosed as iron deficiency anemia.

Remember from our discussion early in the chapter that all trace metals are toxic in excessive amounts. This certainly applies to iron. Iron tablets are so ubiquitous in American households that they present a major hazard to children, acute iron poisoning being a leading cause of childhood poisonings. Some cases have even resulted in death. So when the label says, "Keep out of reach of children," be sure to do so.

More important than treating IDA is making a vigorous attempt to ferret out any underlying diseases of the digestive tract that could have caused the iron loss in the first place. Although a variety of X-ray techniques can evaluate the digestive system, the best method of investigation (also the most expensive and uncomfortable) is gastrointestinal endoscopy. In the "upper GI endoscopy" a fiberoptic flexible endoscope is inserted through the mouth and into the esophagus and parts south. With this procedure, the esophagus, stomach, duodenum, and upper jejunum can be thoroughly examined and biopsied if necessary. The other procedure is the "lower GI endoscopy," in which the scope is passed up the anus to examine the rectum, colon, and lower ileum. The mid portion of the small bowel cannot be easily reached by an endoscope, but fortunately few abnormalities occur in that segment of the gut.

IN SUMMARY

Iron deficiency anemia, one of the most common anemias in the world, can be caused by insufficient iron intake or excessive iron loss, the latter being far more common in the United States. Iron depletion in women of reproductive age is usually caused by menstruation. In all other adult groups, the cause is usually some disease of the digestive tract that must be ferreted out and treated.

4. Vitamin Deficiency Anemias

In Chapter 3 we examined the essential role of iron in the formation of red cells and saw how anemia can result when the body is deficient in it. Although other trace metals, such as cobalt and manganese, are necessary for the production of red cells, iron is by far the most important. Certain vitamins are also required for the production of these cells, including B_{12} (cobalamin), B_6 (pyridoxine), C (ascorbic acid), E (tocopherol), folate (also called folic acid or folacin), riboflavin, pantothenic acid, and thiamin. As with the minerals, some vitamins are more important than others. This chapter is the story of two of those vitamins, B_{12} and folate. Deficiency of either can produce a very severe anemia called *megaloblastic anemia*, which can be defined as *the anemia that occurs as a result of retarded synthesis of DNA in the developing red cells in the marrow*. To understand this definition, we must first look at the marrow to see how red cells develop. Then we need to examine the biochemical nature of DNA and how it is produced. Finally we will correlate the biochemical events in retarded DNA synthesis with the clinical findings in megaloblastic anemia.

INTO THE MARROW

As mentioned in chapter 1, all red blood cells are made in the marrow. The marrow is also the site of production of some (but not all) white cells and all platelets. Red cells in the circulating blood outside the marrow have no nuclei, but their precursors in the marrow, the erythroblasts, must possess nuclei to reproduce. This is because cellular reproduction is impossible unless each new cell has a DNA blueprint to tell it how to develop. The nucleus is the home of that DNA (for more about DNA, see appendix B). Blood cell precursors reproduce by dividing, just as do single-celled organisms like bacteria and protozoa. When one cell divides and becomes two, its DNA is divided almost exactly in half, so that each new daughter cell has half the DNA of its parent. For each of the daughter cells to reproduce in turn, it has to double its DNA content to get back up to the amount of DNA its "mother" had. Therefore, the continual synthesis of new DNA is a fact of life for the dividing erythroblast. If sufficient quantities of DNA cannot be made, then recently divided daughter cells are stymied in their own efforts to reproduce. The marrow then fills up with these aging dowagers who cannot divide. Eventually they die there, having never given rise to new cells.

For reasons that are not clear, another phenomenon experienced by red cell precursors lacking sufficient DNA is failure to mature. Normal red cell precursors cannot go on lingering in the marrow and dividing forever. Eventually a subset of these cells must leave the nest and venture out into a four-month-long dead-end job as a courier in the oxygen transport business. The process by which a red cell precursor transforms from a dividing cell into a circulating one is called *maturation*. Maturation involves three main phenomena: (1) accumulation of hemoglobin, (2) condensation of DNA, and (3) loss of the nucleus.

Assuming plentiful iron stores, accumulation of hemoglobin is presided over by DNA specifically coding for the globin proteins. This DNA transfers its genetic message to RNA by a process called transcription. The RNA (specifically, *messenger RNA*) provides the template upon which amino acids assemble themselves in the proper order to form proteins, including globin. Globin combines with the iron-containing heme to become hemoglobin. For the cell to accumulate hemoglobin, then, there has to be enough messenger RNA upon which to build it, and this means the DNA has to be readily available. For the DNA to be available, it needs to be strung out in long lines in open arrays, like a small amount of cooked spaghetti spread out loosely in a large pot full of water. In such a form, DNA can be easily accessed by the RNA assembling along its length. When enough RNA has been transcribed, DNA is no longer useful and may just as well be put out to pasture: the DNA wads up into a tight ball, resembling drained spaghetti piled on a plate. This phenomenon, condensation of DNA, is readily apparent in routine microscopic examination. What is seen by the hematologist observing the maturation of erythroblasts is the shrinking of the diameter of the nucleus and the transformation of the chromatin (the manifestation of DNA at the microscopic level) from an open, delicate, translucent array to an opaque, hard-looking homogeneous substance.

The final step in red cell maturation is the summary expulsion of the now useless nucleus. The nucleus gets disassembled in the marrow, its molecular components recycled for various uses. For the vast majority of red cells, this final step occurs before the cell leaves the marrow, but a few nucleated cells escape. Their escapade is short-lived, however, as the spleen grabs any nucleated cells on their first pass and plucks out the errant nucleus. The result is that in a patient with normal bone marrow and a normal spleen, nucleated red cells are simply not observed in the circulating blood.

Maturation is mandatory before a red cell can get out of the marrow. If for any reason maturation cannot occur, red cells cannot escape into the bloodstream. This results in two phenomena: (1) anemia, since the circulating red cell population cannot be replenished, and (2) a piling up of erythroblasts in the bone marrow, referred to as ineffective erythropoiesis. For maturation to occur, a sufficient quantity of DNA must be present. Reasoning backwards, it can be concluded that anything keeping DNA from being produced in adequate amounts prevents maturation, which causes anemia and ineffective erythropoiesis. This is the primary abnormality in megaloblastic anemia. Since a deficiency of B_{12} or folate will prevent the synthesis of adequate amounts of DNA, let us take a look at these two vitamins and their roles in this process.

FOLATE

Folate is one of several vitamins required by the body for normal operation. Vitamins are relatively small organic molecules that cannot be manufactured by the body but must be acquired from the food we eat. This means that vitamins are manufactured by the physiologic machinery of the living organisms that make up our food. It is interesting that our bodies, while capable of building thousands of different organic molecules, from the very simple to the enormously complex, are incapable of synthesizing these few (evolution works in mysterious ways). Vitamins as a class of nutrients have widespread applications in every organ system, and folate is no exception. Thus, it is important to keep in mind that, while our emphasis in this book is on anemia, a deficiency of folate has other effects outside the bone marrow.

Unlike iron, which is present in a wide variety of foods, including "junk foods," folate tends to appear in those foods that everyone was told to eat during childhood, but which few unsupervised adults care to consume. The table below gives some examples of the folate content of various foods. Keep in mind that the folate content is given in micrograms, as compared with milligrams for iron. A microgram is $\frac{1}{1,000}$ of a milligram. The conventional Recommended Daily Allowance for folate for nonpregnant adults is 400 micrograms, or 0.4 milligrams. Comparing this with the RDA for iron (10 milligrams for males and nonmenstruating women) shows that, from a standpoint of nutrient mass, we need much more iron than we do folate. Still, since many foods are stingy in folate for the amount of Calories they carry, it is much easier to be deficient in folate than in iron.

Food Item (amount)	Folate Content (micrograms)
liver, beef, fried (3 ounces)	187
asparagus (4 spears)	87
endive, raw, chopped (1 cup)	72
broccoli, boiled (1 small stalk)	70
lettuce, iceberg, raw (1 cup)	61

spinach, raw (1 cup)	58
pizza, pepperoni (1 slice)	53
corn chips (7-ounce bag)	40
chimichanga, fast food (1)	31
beef jerky, one large piece	27
hamburger (1 single-patty, fast-food, plain)	25
beer (12-ounce can/bottle)	21
tomato, raw (1 medium)	18
potato, boiled, no skin (1 medium)	14
doughnut, glazed (1 medium)	13
nachos, fast-food (6–8)	10
chicken, fried, fast-food (2 drumsticks)	9
sausage and biscuit, fast-food (1)	9
grapes, raw (1 cup)	4
frankfurter, beef and pork (1)	2
wine, table (3.5-ounce glass)	1.1
bacon, fried (3 medium slices)	1
distilled spirits (1 jigger)	0

Several nutritional lessons are contained in this brief table:

• Our mothers were right when they told us to eat our green vegetables. The abundance of folate in green, leafy vegetables actually gave this vitamin its name (from the Latin *folium*, "leaf") at the time of its discovery by K. Mitchell in 1941.

• While some junk foods do contain a reasonable amount of folate, they carry too many calories for a given amount of the vitamin. For instance, two 7-ounce bags of corn chips yield just about as much folate as 4 asparagus spears, but the asparagus has only 14 Calories, while the corn chips have over 2,100, enough to maintain a sedentary adult for one day. The significance of this is that the poor, homeless, and unmotivated, while getting by on cheap junk food in terms of caloric intake, may easily become folate-deficient. This is in fact one of the clinical scenarios in which folate deficiency anemia typically rears its head.

• While leafy vegetables are replete with folate, the same may not be true for fruits, such as grapes and tomatoes (yes, tomatoes *are* fruits, regardless of what your cookbooks say). Also, meats, while rich in iron, do not have much folate, especially considering their caloric content.

• Most alcoholic beverages do not contain significant amounts of folate. Beer is an exception, but acquiring from beer alone enough folate to meet one's RDA (400 micrograms), would mean drinking more than three 6-packs per day. Unfortunately, many heavy drinkers get the lion's share of their daily Calories from alcohol; this is one of the reasons that folate deficiency is typically seen in alcoholics, the other being that alcohol itself interferes with the absorption and metabolism of folate, as discussed below.

The absorption of folate in the digestive tract is simple and straightforward. The vitamin is not significantly changed by its trip through the acidic stomach and proceeds to the duodenum and upper jejunum, from which it is readily absorbed into the bloodstream. Folate is stored throughout the body, but it is especially concentrated in the liver. There is always a certain amount of folate circulating in the plasma, and we can easily measure this in the lab by performing a folate level test on a patient's serum. The body's ability to store folate is limited. In fact, full-blown megaloblastic anemia can occur as soon as four months after folate intake is curtailed (the situation with B_{12} is different, as described below).

Regarding megaloblastic anemia, what does folate have to do with making DNA? To answer this question we have to dip into a little biochemistry.

DNA is the abbreviation for "deoxyribonucleic acid." This molecule is composed of a long chain of smaller molecules called *nucleotides*. There are four different nucleotides, thousands of copies of which are linked together in a specific order to make up a gene coding for a specific protein. The nucleotides are adenylate, thymidylate, guanylate, and cytidylate. The body absolutely has to synthesize each of these in order to make DNA. For this discussion, we can forget all the nucleotides except thymidylate, since the body does not need folate to synthesize the other three. To make thymidylate, however, a biochemical step is necessary by which a small part of a molecule, called a methyl group, is transferred from an amino acid to another nucleotide, called uridylate. When this methyl group is transferred to uridylate (and another easy step is performed, involving addition of an oxygen atom to a sugar molecule that is part of uridylate), the uridylate becomes thymidylate, which is then ready for incorporation into DNA.

The methyl group, consisting of a carbon atom surrounded by three hydrogen atoms, is the simplest organic molecule in existence. It seems odd that the body has to resort to a complicated Rube Goldberg-like mechanism to move methyl groups around, but, again, evolution makes no excuses for itself. The transfer of the methyl group to uridylate requires folate. What folate does is to grab the methyl group from two sides, as in a sling. A special tool is required for the moving of methyl groups, because they stick to other molecules so obstinately that it is difficult to get them where they need to go without their becoming permanently bound to the carrier molecule. (Picture yourself trying to throw a sticky piece of tape into the trash, only to have it adhere to your hand. You end up having to use both hands to get rid of it.) Fortunately, we have a molecule that holds on to a methyl group with a two-handed grip just strongly enough to get it where it needs to go without keeping it. If there is no folate, then methyl group transfer cannot occur, DNA cannot be made, and megaloblastic anemia is the result (fig. 4.1).

VITAMIN B₁₂

One of the last vitamins to be discovered (by Karl August Folkers in 1948), B₁₂, or cobalamin, is interesting to both the biochemist and the physician. Sometimes referred to as the most complex molecule in the body that is not just a long repeating chain of simpler units, B₁₂ has such a complicated structure that it was not

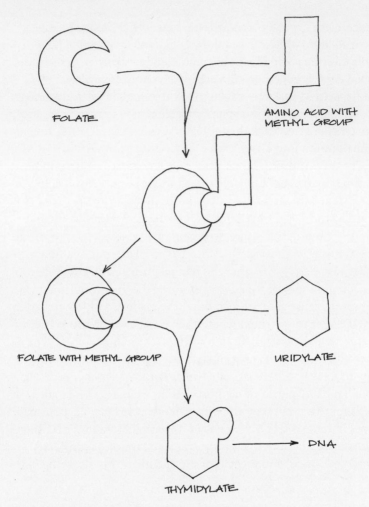

FOLATE

AMINO ACID WITH METHYL GROUP

FOLATE WITH METHYL GROUP

URIDYLATE

DNA

THYMIDYLATE

FIG. 4.1. The role of folate in methyl group transfer.

synthesized until 1971, when the great chemist and Nobel laureate Robert Burns Woodward accomplished that feat. Structurally, B_{12} looks like a molecule "built by a committee"; it consists of a nucleotide (similar to the ones found in DNA) hooked up to a porphyrin-like ring (similar to the one in heme), nestled within which is an atom of the trace metal cobalt (in a position analogous to that of the iron atom in heme). Despite its nucleotide component, B_{12} does not link up in chains like DNA, and despite its heme-like component, it has nothing to do with oxygen transport.

Although absolutely vital to human life, B_{12} is a trace nutrient, and we need only minute daily quantities of it for normal function. The Recommended Daily Allowance for B_{12} is just 3 micrograms. For comparison, the following table shows the RDAs for a sample of other essential nutrients, expressed in microgram units:

Nutrient	Recommended Daily Allowance, male, age 23–50 (micrograms)
vitamin B_{12}	3
folate	400
iron	10,000
vitamin C	60,000
calcium	800,000

The following table shows some representative foods and their B_{12} content.

Food Item (amount)	B_{12} Content (micrograms)
liver, beef, raw (4 ounces)	78
liver, beef, braised (3 ounces)	60
chicken liver, simmered, chopped (1 cup)	27
beef, ribeye, broiled (3 ounces)	2.6
Kellogg's Raisin Bran (1 cup)	1.7
milk, whole (1 cup)	0.9
egg, hard-boiled (1 large)	0.6
frankfurter, beef and pork (1)	0.6
chicken, breaded and fried (1/2 breast)	0.4
bologna, pork (1 medium slice)	0.3
lettuce, iceberg (1 large head)	0
raisins (1.5-ounce box)	0
lentils, boiled (1 cup)	0

Aside from showing that liver has enormous amounts of B_{12}, the table really contains only one simple lesson: that B_{12} is found in animal products only, never in plant products (unless it is artificially added, as in Kellogg's Raisin Bran). A question that comes to mind is this: Since all meat contains B_{12}, and the vegetarian animals we eat must have to make their own (since the plants they eat don't have any B_{12}), is it true that humans are the only animals that cannot synthesize their own B_{12}? The answer is no; in fact *no* animal can make its own B_{12}. So how does the meat we eat come to contain the vitamin? What happens is that, while vegetarian animals cannot make B_{12}, microorganisms living in their digestive systems synthesize it for their own use and have plenty left over to be absorbed by the host. This is an example of symbiosis, or two organisms living together for their mutual benefit. If cattle, for instance, did not provide a home for the microorganisms, the cattle would die of B_{12} deficiency.

The absorption of B_{12} from the digestive tract is more complicated than that of any other nutrient. The vitamin enters the stomach, where it is met by binding proteins called R proteins. The B_{12}-R protein complexes proceed to the duodenum, where the B_{12} is transferred to another protein called *intrinsic factor*. Intrinsic factor is produced by specialized cells, called parietal cells, in the stomach mucosa. Intrinsic factor does not hold onto B_{12} in the acidic environment of the stomach, but as soon as the gastric acid is neutralized in the duodenum, B_{12} and intrinsic factor grab onto each other like long-lost lovers. They are together for the entire trip down the small bowel, because, unlike iron, folate, and just about every other nutrient, B_{12} cannot be absorbed by the duodenum or jejunum. It can be absorbed only by the lower end of the ileum, and this can happen only if it is bound to intrinsic factor. (It is tempting to ask why this is, but those of us in the field of science education have the stock comeback that most of the "why" questions related to evolution are teleological—i. e., having to do with design or purpose—and teleology is not allowed in the Darwinian world. No doubt many turn to the notion of creationism out of pure frustration with the often wacky twists and turns of evolution.)

Now that B_{12} has been absorbed, what does it have to do with making DNA? So far we can only make an educated guess. The role of folate in methyl group transfer is actually more complicated than it appeared to be in the explanation given in the previous section (in fact, *everything* about the body is more complicated than anyone can explain, or even understand). It turns out that not just any kind of folate can pick up and drop off methyl groups—it has to be a special kind, called tetrahydrofolate, or THF. When THF picks up a methyl group, it hangs the group between two nitrogen atoms on its molecule. These nitrogens are denoted by their positions in the THF molecule, namely the 5 and 10 positions, respectively. The THF with its methyl group hooked to the two nitrogens is called N^5,N^{10}-methylene-THF. The normal cycle is for THF to pick up the methyl group, thus becoming N^5,N^{10}-methylene-THF. The latter gives up the methyl group to uridylate (changing it to thymidylate), and the N^5,N^{10}-methylene-THF, now bereft of the methyl group, becomes THF again. This should go on ad infinitum, but the problem is that THF, like some other carriers we have met (hemoglobin, for instance) is a rather fragile molecule. In enduring the vicissitudes of life in a crowded environment of unfriendly biomolecules, a certain percentage of N^5,N^{10}-methyl-THF will suffer the detachment of its methyl group from one of the nitrogens holding it. The resulting molecule still has its methyl group hanging on by its bond with the other nitrogen. This molecule is called N^5-methyl-THF. The methyl group on N^5-methyl-THF is held too strongly by its single bond to be easily given up to uridylate. The N^5-methyl-THF, then, is perfectly content to go right on as it is, never to participate in methyl group transfer again. This means not only that the methyl group does not get transferred, but that the folate molecule it is hooked to will never again be available to do its job. This scenario is called, somewhat melodramatically, the folate trap (fig. 4.2). Once again, however, evolution has provided a way out: an enzyme called methyltransferase.

Enzymes are protein molecules that speed up chemical reactions. From a biological standpoint, without the help of an enzyme almost every reaction in a living organism would proceed so slowly that it might as well not happen at all. Accordingly, enzymes collectively represent the mechanism by which just about all biochemical reactions occur. In the case of methyltransferase, the reaction is the removal of the methyl group from N5-methyl-THF, yielding THF, which jumps right back into the fray by picking up methyl groups and transferring them to uridylate. Happy ending? Well, it

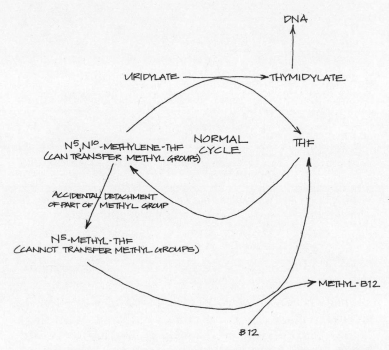

FIG. 4.2. The folate trap. In the absence of B_{12}, N5-methyl-THF accumulates, and there is insufficient THF for participation in methyl group transfer.

is not quite that simple. By definition, enzymes are catalysts, and catalysts are not chemically altered in the reactions they participate in. Methyltransferase, therefore, cannot leave the playing field in possession of its trophy, the methyl group it took from N5-methyl-THF. It has to give the methyl group to some other molecule, and the only one that fits the bill is B_{12}. In the methyltransferase reaction, then, B_{12} picks up the methyl group from methyltransferase, so that the latter can go on about its business. The B_{12} molecule itself, now called methyl-B_{12}, has no trouble giving up its methyl group to an obliging amino acid, thus recycling B_{12} for use in further reactions.

SUMMARY OF NORMAL FOLATE AND B_{12} FUNCTION

The function of folate is to transfer methyl groups to uridylate, forming thymidylate, from which DNA is made. Some folate molecules are inactivated when they lose half their grip on the methyl groups they carry. The function of B_{12} is to help an enzyme clear that methyl group off the folate molecule, so that the latter becomes functional again. The significance of all this is that if either B_{12} or folate is not present in sufficient quantities, DNA cannot be made. If DNA cannot be made, the reproduction and maturation of red cell precursors stalls in the marrow, causing anemia and ineffective erythropoiesis.

Now that we have covered the roles of folate and B_{12} in normal physiology, we will look at how deficiencies occur.

FOLATE DEFICIENCY

There are several ways in which the body can become deficient in folate.

(1) *Dietary deficiency*. In chapter 3 we saw that inadequate diet alone was not likely to result in iron deficiency. Folate is a different story. Because it is so easy to obtain Calories sufficient

to sustain life from a variety of cheap, junk foods that do not contain much folate, deficiency of the vitamin is very common in the diets of poor people and of those who have lost the motivation to take good care of themselves. Accordingly, the most common cause of folate deficiency is malnutrition, and the persons most likely to suffer from that come from the neglected, poor, demented, or alcoholic segments of society.

(2) *Malabsorption.* We saw in chapter 3 how diseases of the GI tract can cause malabsorption of iron; the same situations apply to folate.

(3) *Increased requirement for folate.* A high rate of cellular reproduction calls for a large amount of folate to allow sufficient DNA synthesis for cell division. The time of life in which cell division is the greatest is infancy. Pound for pound, an infant needs 5 to 10 times the amount of folate that an adult does. This daily folate requirement turns out to be approximately the amount found in 1 liter (1.06 quart) of mother's milk. This is a fairly tall order, even for the most fecund breast, so the baby is at best living on the edge of folate imbalance. Infants are, therefore, prime candidates for folate deficiency.

Since the high rate of cellular growth in the developing child is also present in the developing fetus, pregnant women are very susceptible to folate deficiency. This is especially true of women who have not had the advantage of a well-balanced diet before and during pregnancy. There is a second reason why women should be sure to get adequate folate intake during pregnancy: it has been shown recently that many cases of a certain type of severe fetal deformity, called neural tube defects, can be prevented by adequate folate intake.

States of increased cellular division may occur in certain disease states, including cancer, and, as we shall see in chapter 5, hemolytic anemias. For this reason, it is especially important for patients with these diseases to maintain a healthy folate intake.

(4) *Interference with folate metabolism.* Various drugs, including anticancer drugs, alcohol, and even the anesthetic gas nitrous oxide, interfere with the work of folate in DNA synthesis.

B$_{12}$ DEFICIENCY

Deficiency of B$_{12}$, like that of folate, can arise as the result of several underlying physiological disturbances, but the scenarios involving the two vitamins are different.

(1) *Dietary deficiency.* Vitamin B$_{12}$ is so prevalent in animal products that it is almost impossible for someone to develop a deficiency through diet alone. Only those individuals who adhere to strict vegetarianism with religious fervor can suffer this fate. Moreover, only those vegetarians who do not eat milk and eggs (called vegans) stand to become B$_{12}$ deficient. Even in this small group, dietary B$_{12}$ deficiency is rare, because the body is normally so good at holding on to whatever B$_{12}$ has already been acquired for long periods of time (3 to 5 years). On the other hand, breast-fed babies of vegan women are much more at risk than their mothers and can develop megaloblastic anemia in infancy. Unfortunately, as we will see later in the discussion of the nonhematological role of B$_{12}$ in physiology, these babies may develop permanent neurological damage before the problem can be diagnosed.

(2) *Pernicious anemia.* Occupying a special place in the halls of hematological history, pernicious anemia, or PA, was the subject of the medical study that first brought us into the molecular age of hematology. It is also one of only two blood diseases (the other being malaria) for which its investigators were awarded a Nobel Prize. The conquest of PA, once considered invariably fatal (the word "pernicious" means "deadly"), was one of the great victories for early twentieth century medical science.

Briefly defined, *pernicious anemia is the condition that results from failure to absorb vitamin B$_{12}$, resulting from unavailability of intrinsic factor (IF), resulting from destruction of IF and the cells that produce it.* The sequence of pathophysiological phenomena is (a) destruction of IF-producing cells in the stomach, accompanied by neutralization of whatever IF the remaining cells produce, (b) failure of B$_{12}$ to be bound to IF in the duodenum, (c) failure of unbound B$_{12}$ to be absorbed in the lower ileum, (d) B_{12} deficiency in the marrow, and (e) megaloblastic anemia. The key event in the genesis of PA, then, is something that causes destruction of gastric mucosal cells and neutralization of IF. The true identity of the villain of this story is unknown, but one possibility is autoantibodies, the effectors of the class of conditions collectively called *autoimmune diseases*.

In autoimmune diseases, the body's immune system turns against its own tissues. Commonly recognized autoimmune diseases are systemic lupus erythematosus, scleroderma, rheumatoid arthritis, and Hashimoto's thyroiditis. Others exist as well, and it is possible that a whole host of diseases of unknown cause may turn out to be autoimmune. No one knows what goads the immune system into attacking the body's own tissues, although it is possible that some heretofore unknown infectious microorganism could get the ball rolling and start the body on a long downhill course of self-destruction. In the case of pernicious anemia, the autoantibodies are directed against the IF-secreting parietal cells in the gastric mucosa, which they destroy, and against intrinsic factor, which they neutralize. It should be noted that, although the autoantibodies are detectable in many PA patients, it is not clear if such antibodies are the *cause* or *result* of the disease.

Pernicious anemia is classically considered a disease of elderly men and women of Scandinavian or other northern European descent. Although advanced age certainly is a factor, PA can occur in any racial or ethnic group.

(3) *Surgical removal of the stomach*, or *gastrectomy*. This procedure for cancer or severe ulcer disease removes some or all of the cells that produce intrinsic factor. Therefore, B_{12} deficiency may eventually develop if the patient does not receive B_{12} supplements.

(4) *Malabsorption*. Conditions similar to those which cause folate or iron deficiency can also cause B_{12} deficiency. Because the B_{12}-IF complex is absorbed only in the lower ileum, diseases that affect this area of the gut can cause B_{12} deficiency. Of particular note is Crohn's disease, a chronic inflammatory condition of

unknown cause that tends to affect this particular segment of the digestive tract.

(5) *Competition.* This circumstance is an unusual cause of B_{12} deficiency. The competition may take the form of a particular parasite called the fish tapeworm or of the overgrowth of normal intestinal bacteria following bowel surgery and in cases of anatomic deformities of the intestines. In either case, dietary B_{12} is consumed by the competitors, leaving insufficient amounts for the host.

SYMPTOMS OF MEGALOBLASTIC ANEMIA

A person with megaloblastic anemia will complain of some or all of the symptoms of anemia in general. According to our cytometric classification of anemia (introduced in chapter 2), this is a *macrocytic, normochromic anemia.* In other words, the red cells in the peripheral blood are abnormally large, but their individual concentration of hemoglobin is normal. Of course, for the whole-blood hemoglobin to be low (thus conforming to our clinical definition of anemia), the RBC count has to be disproportionately low to yield the high mean corpuscular volume (MCV) that defines macrocytic anemia. The reason that red cells in megaloblastic anemias are so large is that, while they are waiting in the marrow for the slowed-down maturation of their nuclei to be completed, they continue to synthesize hemoglobin at a normal rate (remember, there is plenty of iron for heme, and plenty of RNA for translation of globin proteins, so hemoglobin production goes on as if nothing else is happening). Since the red cells are sitting in the marrow longer than normal and getting fatter with hemoglobin all the time, when (and if) they finally get out into the bloodstream, they are bloated monstrosities with volumes up to one and a half times what is normal. While still in the marrow, the nucleated red cell precursors (erythroblasts) are also larger than normal—thus the terms megaloblast ("big blast"), and megaloblastic anemia.

Because folate and B₁₂ are required for the proper proliferation of all DNA-requiring cells in the body, various other findings are present in a person with megaloblastic anemia. For one thing, the tongue is smooth and shiny, as it is when there is iron deficiency. The precursors of white cells and platelets in the marrow also suffer retarded maturation, resulting in abnormally low white blood cell counts and platelet counts. Even the cells lining the cervix of the uterus are affected; their large size may fool the examiner of a woman's Pap smear into thinking that a precancerous condition exists (in fact, there is nothing precancerous about megaloblastic anemia).

In addition to the clinical findings common to megaloblastic anemias caused by deficiency of either B₁₂ or folate, B₁₂-deficient persons suffer from an additional set of abnormalities not seen in those with folate deficiency: neurological symptoms. Vitamin B₁₂ has an important nonhematological role in the maintenance of nerve cells (neurons) that make up the brain, spinal cord, and peripheral nerves. In particular, B₁₂ is necessary for the construction and/or maintenance of the sheath of fatty material, called myelin, that surrounds the long wire-like processes of neurons, called axons. If the myelin is defective, the ability of the cell to carry signal impulses is diminished. This is true of both sensory impulses (those that carry information to the brain) and motor impulses (which carry signals from the brain telling muscles to contract in a coordinated fashion). Because the abnormality affects both the sensory and motor systems, the term used to describe the neurological condition in those with B₁₂ deficiency is combined systems disease.

Combined systems disease becomes clinically apparent first in the parts of the body subserved by the longest axons, the extremities (arms and legs). Individuals typically complain of numbness or "pins-and-needles" discomfort in the fingers and toes and may become concerned that they are clumsy in performing tasks requiring manual dexterity. Eventually the patient has difficulty in walking and may indeed become essentially paralyzed. In the physical examination, the doctor (using a vibrating tuning fork held against the person's skin), finds a deficiency in the perception of vibration. Diminished proprioception, or the inability to tell without looking, for instance, which way one's toes or fingers are pointing, is another early finding. Patients may also develop aberrant behavior and exhibit symptoms of mental illness. A very rare, extreme manifestation of this tendency is frank schizophrenic behavior, referred to as megaloblastic madness.

Knowledge of the clinical features of combined systems disease is extremely important to the primary care physician, because failure to recognize and treat it at an early stage can result in permanent disability. Even with early treatment, the damage already done to the nervous system is usually irreversible. Compounding the diagnostic problem is the fact that combined systems disease may become well established before any significant degree of anemia is manifest.

Modern laboratory medicine has given us inexpensive and readily available tests for the definitive diagnosis of megaloblastic anemias. In the typical sequence of clinical events, (1) the routine complete blood count (CBC) shows macrocytic, normochromic anemia, (2) serum B_{12} and folate levels are ordered, and (3) if one or both levels are low the person is given definitive B_{12} or folate replacement treatment.

In the case of B_{12} deficiency, it is sometimes desirable to determine exactly how the deficiency occurred. The Schilling test is classically used for this purpose; it is usually not necessary for accurate diagnosis, but it may be useful in more complex or confusing cases. In this test, a person is given an oral dose of B_{12}, the cobalt atom of which is radioactive, so that the B_{12} molecule is labeled with radioactivity that can be detected in a radiation counter. In a normal person, the radiolabeled B_{12} is absorbed by the process described above. It is then excreted in the urine, which is measured for radioactivity to confirm the presence of the labelled B_{12}. In a patient with PA or malabsorption, the B_{12} will not be absorbed, so the urine will not contain the expected amount of labelled B_{12}. When this is the case, the next step is to give the patient another dose of radiolabeled B_{12}, this time with an oral dose of intrinsic factor. In a patient with PA, the added IF should correct the problem, the B_{12} is absorbed, and the label is detected in the urine. If the cause of B_{12} deficiency is malabsorption, as from Crohn's disease, then the IF will not correct the problem, and the label will not be excreted.

TREATMENT OF MEGALOBLASTIC ANEMIA

The treatment of megaloblastic anemia is simply replacement of the vitamin in which the person is deficient. If the cause of the deficiency is dietary (much more common with folate than with B_{12}), then oral replacement therapy is necessary. If the deficiency is due to failure to absorb the nutrient (as in pernicious anemia), then obviously oral therapy will have no effect, and injections are required. Some absorption problems can be permanently corrected surgically or with other treatment, but PA has no cure; the person will require B_{12} injections for life.

The initial treatment for pernicious anemia involves daily intramuscular injections of as much as 1,000 micrograms of B_{12}, the red-colored solution so familiar to physicians of the old days, who gave a totally unnecessary shot of the crimson vitamin to any elderly patient who came in with any complaint. This is a huge dose, representing the B_{12} content of 72 pounds of rib-eye steak. Fortunately, the body's storage pools of B_{12} are replenished rapidly, and eventually the injections are reduced to a 1,000-microgram dose once a month.

Folate-deficient persons often belong to the segment of humanity swept under society's rug, and no amount of medical knowledge can eliminate conditions of poverty, neglect, alcoholism, or drug addiction. In this disease, as with many others outside the realm of hematology, social problems may prove far more daunting than medical ones.

Both folate and B_{12} deficiency respond dramatically to replacement therapy. Sometimes a nutritionally folate-deficient person will respond just to eating a balanced hospital meal. The hematological lab values in such a case will begin to correct themselves before the proper diagnosis is made, producing a confusing clinical picture. Those with pernicious anemia in particular may feel so good within hours of beginning treatment that they can be described as "euphoric." Measurable reversions of hematologic lab values back toward the normal occur within hours, in contrast to the analogous situation with iron deficiency anemia, which takes weeks to correct.

IN SUMMARY

The vitamins B_{12} and folate are necessary for red cell precursors to proliferate and mature in the marrow. If either vitamin is deficient, the marrow fills up with red cell precursors (a condition known as ineffective erythropoiesis), and the few cells that are released into the bloodstream are too big (macrocytic, normochromic anemia). Folate deficiency is seen in poorly nourished individuals, pregnant women, and alcoholics. Deficiency of B_{12} is usually caused by failure to absorb the vitamin in the digestive tract, due to the destruction of the cells in the stomach that produce intrinsic factor, a necessary component for the absorption of B_{12}. This is called pernicious anemia. Both folate and B_{12} deficiency anemias can be corrected by replacement therapy with the appropriate vitamin, but in B_{12} deficiency there may be uncorrectable and disabling permanent neurological damage.

The following table shows expected lab results in patients with megaloblastic anemias:

Test	Result in Folate Deficiency	Result in B_{12} Deficiency
hemoglobin	low	low
MCV	high	high
MCHC	normal	normal
serum folate	low	normal
serum B_{12}	normal	low

In this and the previous chapter, we have dealt with deficiency diseases that keep the marrow from producing sufficient circulating red cell mass. We will now examine diseases in which the marrow function is totally normal, but anemia results anyway.

5. Hemolytic Anemias

Briefly defined, hemolytic anemias are *those anemias that result from abnormally shortened red cell life span*. Any condition in which there is shortened RBC life span is termed *hemolysis* (literally "destruction of blood"). In these cases, the marrow is perfectly normal and in fact really gets to showcase its talents in turning out prodigious numbers of red cells. Anemia occurs because circulating red cells are destroyed faster than even a marrow revved up to full steam can replace them. The accelerated destruction of red cells can be caused either by a problem with the makeup of the red cell itself or by a physiological environment inimical to the red cell. In this chapter, we will cover first the normal events in the aging and death of red cells, then the clinical diagnosis of hemolytic anemia in general, and finally the various specific hemolytic anemias.

RED CELLS: CRABBED AGE AND YOUTH

Regarding reproduction, there are two types of cells in the human body: those that replace themselves, and those that don't. The latter category includes neurons, muscle cells (including heart cells), bone cells, cartilage cells, and connective tissue cells; by the time we reach full adult size we have all of these that we will ever need. Some, such as bone, cartilage, and connective tissue cells, are capable of proliferating to rebuild damaged areas, as in wound healing with scar formation or fracture healing following a broken bone. Other cells in this category, such as neurons and muscle cells, are not capable of proliferating to repair damage (although they can regrow parts of themselves lost to injury).

The other type of cells, those that replace themselves, do not live as long as the whole organism. Their life span is a fraction of the life span of the host. Most of these cells fall into one of two categories: those which cover surfaces of the body (the epithelial cells) and blood cells. Although there may seem to be little similarity between these types of cells, what they do have in common is that they are *easy to lose*. In the case of epithelial cells, the mere interaction with a traumatic foreign environment, either internal (as with the digestive tract mucosa) or external (as with the skin), results in wear and tear that causes wholesale loss of cells, which have to be replaced by a reserve of proliferating cells. In the case of blood cells, most of the white cells and all of the platelets are used up fighting invaders and stopping bleeding, respectively. Red cells are lost through even the most insignificant cuts, scrapes, bruises, and nosebleeds. The solution lies in the constant replacement of the short-lived cells.

Red cells are released by the marrow after a maturation period of about five days (a process described in chapter 4). For one day after their release they continue to display a vestige of their youthful days in the marrow, a substance called *reticulum*. Reticulum represents balled-up, now useless RNA that was originally involved in the translation of globin protein to make hemoglobin. This substance is easily observed through routine microscopy, if the blood smear has been colored with a special stain called a supravital dye. Such stained cells, called *reticulocytes*, can be counted, and the proportion of these to other red cells is called the *reticulocyte count*. The normal reticulocyte count (or "retic count") is between 0.5 and 1.5 percent. This seems like an insignificant number, but, as we shall see later, the retic count is one of the most important lab tests in the diagnosis of hemolytic anemia.

After the first day in the circulation, the reticulocytes have lost all their reticulum and are now indistinguishable from all the other RBCs in the blood. After circulating for about 120 days, it is time for the red cell's days to end. Somehow, for reasons that are unknown, the body system that functions as the red cell's grim reaper, the *reticuloendothelial system* (RES), captures the aged cell and destroys it. The RES consists of a variety of tissues and organs in the body, including the spleen, the liver, and even the bone marrow itself. Each of these organs contains cavern-like spaces, called *sinusoids*, which are lined by special cells called *fixed phagocytes* (from Greek roots meaning "eater cells"). The function of the fixed phagocytes, and their more mobile cousins, the *macrophages*, is to engulf the obsolete red cells, destroy them, and recycle their components. The molecular mechanisms by which certain red cell components are recycled are relevant to the clinical investigation of anemia, so let us briefly revisit biochemistry.

Most of the red cell consists of hemoglobin suspended in a watery medium, so we need only to consider how hemoglobin is broken down and recycled. First, heme is removed from globin. Globin is nothing more than a regular old protein, which the body breaks down every day. It, like all other recycled proteins, is broken down to its constituent amino acids, which are then transported in the plasma to the liver and other organs (with some going back to the marrow, of course, to make more globin). The amino acids can then be reassembled along DNA-programmed messenger RNA templates to make whatever proteins the body needs at the time. The way heme is handled is very special, however. The heme molecule is a ring-shaped structure with an atom of iron loosely held in the center of the ring. The iron is removed, bound to plasma proteins, transported back to the marrow, and held in storage; developing red cells can draw from it to make their own hemoglobin. At the same time the iron is removed from heme, the organic, porphyrin-like ring structure is dealt with. Unlike iron and globin, the iron-less ring is not recycled but excreted (fig. 5.1). The means by which the body does this is complex. First, the ring structure is cleaved at a single point, yielding an open ring (which is of course no longer a ring at all). This new molecule is called biliverdin. In the process of breakage of the ring, one molecule of carbon monoxide is released into the body. The fact that a natural metabolic phenomenon produces a deadly gas is excellent rebuttal to those individuals who maintain that whatever is "natural" is good for you, and whatever is "artificial" is bad. Of course, the reason that we all don't die of carbon monoxide poisoning before birth is that the concentration of the toxin never gets high enough to cause any adverse effects.

The biliverdin, while still in the cells of the reticuloendothelial system, undergoes a conversion to a substance called *bilirubin*. In terms of its physical appearance, bilirubin is yellow in low concentrations and green in high ones. Accumulation of abnormal amounts of bilirubin in tissues is called *jaundice* (*jaune* is French for "yellow"). Jaundice is a clinical sign readily recognized at early stages by the experienced physician and at late stages by anyone. For some reason, patients themselves seem unable to see their own jaundice in the mirror until they are severely affected. The measurement of bilirubin in serum is a routine clinical lab test. The normal range for serum bilirubin is anything less than about 1.4 milligrams per deciliter. As we shall see later, jaundice is a sign of hemolytic anemia, but it is more commonly seen in diseases of the liver and bile ducts.

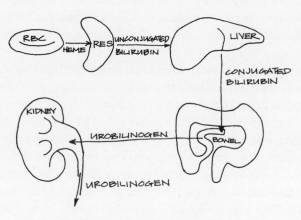

FIG. 5.1. The breakdown and excretion of heme.

Bilirubin leaves the RES bound to a plasma protein called albumin. This type of bilirubin is measured in the lab as something called indirect bilirubin. The indirect bilirubin is dropped off in the liver for excretion. The liver treats bilirubin in the same way it treats numerous other drugs and toxins it gets rid of, which is by attaching to it two molecules of a sugar-like substance called glucuronic acid. The resulting molecule is called bilirubin diglucuronide. The liver summarily dumps the bilirubin diglucuronide, also called conjugated bilirubin, into the bile ducts that run from the liver and ultimately coalesce into one duct, the common bile duct, which empties its contents out into the duodenum. The intense color of concentrated bilirubin is what gives bile its familiar green color. Moreover, it is the bile that makes normal feces yellowish-brown; feces without any bile is actually gray (gray stool being one of the symptoms of bile duct obstruction and of some liver diseases).

Now that the bilirubin has been flushed into the sewer of the body, one might think that it need not be considered further, but the story is not yet over. The conjugated bilirubin remains pretty much unaltered and only minimally absorbed through its long journey down the small bowel. The meager amount that gets absorbed back into the bloodstream is measurable in the serum as direct bilirubin (normal range, less than 0.4 milligrams per deciliter). Once the unabsorbed conjugated bilirubin gets to the last part of the ileum and into the colon, however, it is once again metabolized. This time the normal colonic bacteria are the ones doing the work, namely, stripping the two glucuronides off the bilirubin molecule, so that it is once again unconjugated, as it was before being picked up by the liver. In addition, the bacteria convert the colored bilirubin molecules into a class of related colorless substances collectively called urobilinogen. Most of the urobilinogen is excreted in the feces, but some is actually reabsorbed into the bloodstream. The body is not stuck with it forever, though, because the second excretory system in the body, headed by the kidneys, quickly filters the urobilinogen into the urine. Urobilinogen, being colorless, does not give urine its amber color, which is due to unrelated substances called urochromes. Urobilinogen is important clinically, because it can be measured in the routine urinalysis by means of a simple dipstick test.

There is one more item to consider before moving on to hemolytic anemia proper, and that is the not-quite-perfect table manners of the reticuloendothelial system. It seems that when an RES cell gobbles up a red cell, a few crumbs may be spilled. This means that a very small amount of hemoglobin escapes the maw of the macrophage to end up circulating free in the plasma. From a conservation standpoint, this is bad news, because hemoglobin circulating free in the plasma is very unstable. In fact, once liberated from the comfortable confines of the red cell, hemoglobin breaks in half. The halves are too small to escape being filtered by the kidney, so this hemoglobin, complete with its precious iron, is flushed out of the body in the urine. Once again, however, evolution has come up with a solution. The figurative napkin-in-the-lap to catch the hemoglobin crumbs is a normal plasma protein called *haptoglobin*. Haptoglobin just floats around in the plasma doing nothing until it encounters a molecule of hemoglobin, at which time the haptoglobin grabs fiercely onto the hemoglobin. The combined *haptoglobin-hemoglobin complex* is much too big to be filtered into the urine by the kidneys, so hemoglobin and its iron are conserved. The complex can then take a leisurely trip via the bloodstream back to the RES, where it is disassembled and recycled, as in the above description.

If hemolysis is brisk enough, so much hemoglobin is spilled into the plasma that all the haptoglobin is used up. In such instances, free hemoglobin (after its molecules spontaneously break in two) is filtered by the kidneys and is summarily excreted in the urine. This is called *hemoglobinuria*. If severe enough, hemoglobinuria can be visible to the naked eye as red-colored urine. Lesser degrees of hemoglobinuria may not be visible, but the simple dipstick urinalysis can detect it.

DIAGNOSING HEMOLYTIC ANEMIA

In a typical clinical scenario, a person shows signs and symptoms of anemia, and the diagnosis is confirmed by a low hemoglobin. Hemolytic anemias are usually *normocytic, normochromic*, meaning that the average red cell is of normal size and contains a normal concentration of hemoglobin, which is not surprising, because the red cell production facility is completely normal. The doctor then makes the diagnosis of normochromic, normocytic anemia; however, many anemias fall into this category. The first question to ask is whether the anemia is due to lowered cell production (hyporegenerative anemia) or shortened red cell life span (hemolytic anemia). This distinction is made by means of one or more laboratory tests:

(1) *Reticulocyte count*. The retic count is the most important test in the initial classification of a normocytic anemia. In hemolytic anemias, the marrow kicks into high gear and increases the rate of production of red cells severalfold. In addition, like the famed ninety-day wonders of World War II, red cells are kicked out into the bloodstream before they are fully mature, resulting in reticulocytes that are identifiable as such for two or three days instead of one. The result is that the proportion of reticulocytes in the blood rises severalfold above the normal level of less than 1.5 percent. In fact, in a severe case of hemolytic anemia, the retic count may be as high as 20 percent.

Conversely, in hyporegenerative normocytic anemias, the reticulocyte is not elevated and may even be low. The retic count is highly reliable, inexpensive, and easily done in even the most primitively equipped laboratories. Amazingly, considering its clinical value and technical feasibility, many physicians fail to make use of the reticulocyte count. In my opinion, the failure to order a retic count is the most common mistake made by physicians in the assessment of anemia.

As great as it is, the retic count is not a perfect test. For one thing, an elevated retic count is not diagnostic of hemolytic anemia. As we saw in chapter 4, the response of megaloblastic anemias to replacement therapy is often dramatic. This response is characterized by the tremendously accelerated production of red cells by the marrow, which is manifested as an elevated retic count. Some early cases of iron deficiency may not yet show the characteristic microcytosis of the fully developed case. Moreover, since iron deficiency often results from bleeding episodes, and bleeding tends to stimulate a reticulocyte response, even iron deficiency anemia can masquerade as a hemolytic anemia. Fortunately, for these confusing cases we have other tests designed to detect accelerated RBC destruction more directly. The remaining tests fall into this category.

(2) *Blood smear examination.* In some types of hemolytic anemia (such as microangiopathic hemolytic anemia, discussed below), the shape of the red cells is abnormal. The appearance of the red cell is easily assessed through a peripheral smear examination. A drop of blood is placed on a glass microscope slide, and the edge of another slide is drawn into the drop. Just before the drop has spread over the interface between the edge of the second slide and the surface of the first slide, the second slide is smartly scraped over the length of the first. The result is a flame-shaped smear on the first slide. The end of the smear at which the blood was first dropped is too thick to examine, but out toward the feathered edge at the opposite end, the smear is just thin enough to allow the cells to be seen in all their individual glory. The technique of making smears is somewhat more difficult than it sounds, and laboratorians must get quite a bit of practice and critical review to become proficient.

Of course, nothing of interest can be seen on an unstained smear. Routinely, one of the Romanowsky stains (see chapter 1), usually the Wright stain, is employed to make the cells visible (remember that reticulocytes need special supravital dyes to be visible as such; retics cannot be distinguished from other red cells on the Wright stain).

The next step is to put the slide under a microscope and examine it; this is usually done at two levels of magnification,

100X and 1000X. The low power is for screening the smear for rare abnormal cells, and the high one for discerning the details of the cells found by screening. In the case of hemolytic anemias, the examiner looks for evidence that the cells have been injured in the circulation, as in microangiopathic hemolytic anemias, and for the presence of abnormal inclusions in the red cells, as would be seen in some other types of hemolytic anemia. With rare exceptions, the only people truly qualified to evaluate a blood smear thoroughly are hematologists (medical or pediatric subspecialists who have undertaken one or more years of fellowship training) and laboratorians (pathologists, medical technologists, and medical laboratory technicians).

(3) *Serum bilirubin level.* Because of the accelerated destruction of red cells in hemolytic anemia, heme is broken down more rapidly. Unconjugated bilirubin (or indirect bilirubin, as it is called in the lab) accumulates in the plasma, because the cellular machinery in the liver that normally collects, conjugates, and excretes it is overwhelmed. The level of bilirubin is measured in serum with a very simple routine test available in any hospital or reference lab. If the level of bilirubin in the plasma is high enough (about 2 milligrams per deciliter), then the doctor may notice clinical jaundice. (Actually, the recognition of jaundice at this low level of bilirubin presumes excellent lighting conditions, equivalent to bright sunlight outdoors.) In hemolytic anemias where the liver function is normal, the serum bilirubin rarely exceeds 7 milligrams per deciliter. Much higher levels of bilirubin (up to 50 milligrams per deciliter) may be observed in patients with diseases of the liver or bile ducts.

Because jaundice is seen not only in hemolytic anemias but also in liver and bile duct disease, the doctor is interested in knowing the relative proportions of conjugated (direct) and unconjugated (indirect) bilirubin in the serum. In liver and biliary tract disease, there is more conjugated than unconjugated bilirubin in the serum, while in hemolytic anemia, the reverse is true. Accordingly, the serum bilirubin test typically yields three results: total, indirect, and direct bilirubin.

(4) *Urine urobilinogen.* This is part of the routine urinalysis dipstick test that can be performed in any doctor's office or lab. In the hemolytic state, the liver churns out conjugated bilirubin at full tilt. Some of this is eventually converted to urobilinogen by bowel bacteria, reabsorbed, and excreted in the urine, where increased amounts are detected by the dipstick test.

(5) *Serum haptoglobin level.* Because of the sloppy spilling of hemoglobin by the RES while it disposes of red cells, in times of brisk hemolysis more hemoglobin is spilled. This is quickly complexed to haptoglobin and cleared from the plasma by the RES. If hemolysis is rapid enough, all of the haptoglobin is used up, and it is undetectable in the serum by a lab test. Therefore, the serum haptoglobin can be used as a measure of hemolysis—the lower the serum haptoglobin, the worse the hemolysis.

(6) *Urine hemoglobin.* The kidneys are so good at keeping red cells from falling out of the blood vessels that no hemoglobin is detectable in normal urine. The routine dipstick urinalysis can detect any hemoglobin that escapes into the urine in the course of brisk hemolysis. A positive hemoglobin test by dipstick is not diagnostic for hemoglobinuria, however, since any of a number of conditions, from simple urinary tract infections to kidney or bladder cancer, can cause blood in the urine.

SPECIFIC HEMOLYTIC ANEMIAS

After the doctor determines that a person has normocytic, normochromic anemia, and then that it is a hemolytic anemia, the next challenge is to ascertain the cause. In some cases this can be done with great exactitude, essentially at the molecular level; in others, the mechanism may remain vague. Either way, this determination dictates how the anemic person will be treated. Each of the following sections covers one of the major types of hemolytic anemia, including an explanation of how the red cells are destroyed, how the disease is clinically diagnosed, and the strategy for treatment.

Microangiopathic hemolytic anemias

This class of hemolytic anemia is a lot more straightforward than its long name would suggest. Breaking the word down (*micro,* "small"; *angio,* "vessel"; *pathic,* "causing disease"), we get "a hemolytic anemia caused by disease in the small (blood) vessels." The most straightforward way to destroy red cells is just to beat them up; they are simply bags of liquid, like water balloons, and are subject to destruction by any sufficiently strong compressive or shearing force. The normal shape of the red cells affords their easy passage through even the tiny capillaries, which are wide enough to allow red cells to get through in single file. If there is an obstruction in the small vessels, however, the red cells will either clog up behind it or be torn apart while trying to squeeze through. In several conditions, formation of intravascular obstructions is just big enough to tear up the red cells without stopping the flow of blood altogether. The obstructions are composed of the protein that makes up a normal blood clot. This protein is called fibrin, and the obstruction it forms is called a fibrin clot. Red cells are sheared apart, or "clotheslined," when forced across the fibrin clot. Many of the cells are totally destroyed by this process, but some of them desperately try to reassemble themselves and regain their cellular competence. These abnormally shaped cells can be easily seen on the blood smear. Typically having the shape of an American soldier's steel helmet, they are called *helmet cells,* the medical name being *schizocytes* (literally, "broken cells"). This is one reason why it is so important to examine a blood smear in cases of suspected hemolytic anemia.

In several diseases there is extensive abnormal formation of fibrin clots throughout the body, leading to microangiopathic hemolytic anemia:

(1) *Disseminated intravascular coagulopathy* (DIC). DIC is not a disease in itself, but is a common complication of a fairly large variety of other serious acute diseases. In DIC, there is an abnormal and inappropriate activation of the blood clotting system, so that clots form within normal blood vessels (clots

usually form only in the immediate vicinity of an injured vessel). Red cells get hung on the clots and are sheared apart. In the process of forming clots, fibrinogen (the plasma protein that is converted to fibrin in the formation of clots) is used up and is therefore no longer available to form normal clots at any sites of vessel injury. Other clotting proteins and platelets are used up as well, so they are not available either. When circulating levels of platelets and clotting proteins are sufficiently low, the normal clotting system does not work, and abnormal bleeding occurs. This is paradoxical, since the whole DIC process begins with abnormal clotting, and the problem which develops is abnormal bleeding. The abnormal fibrin clots not only use up platelets and coagulation factors, but also interfere with blood supply to vital organs. The kidneys are especially sensitive to loss of blood flow, so another complication of DIC is acute renal failure.

DIC was first discovered in women suffering from a variety of obstetrical complications, but it is now seen more commonly in elderly people with severe bacterial infections. The list of diseases that cause DIC is long, but the main thing to remember about it is that DIC can occur as a result of just about any disease that makes the patient severely and acutely ill.

In planning the treatment of a patient with DIC, the doctor is in a classic "between a rock and a hard place" predicament. To stop the abnormal clotting, the patient can be given heparin, a drug that reliably stops that process. The problem is that the person is already bleeding because all the clotting proteins and platelets have been used up, and heparin would only inactivate whatever feeble amount of clotting proteins he or she has. The doctor might try to stop the bleeding by replacing the depleted platelets and clotting proteins with transfusions; the problem here is that it adds fuel to the fire of abnormal clotting that started the whole business. What can give the doctor hope is that DIC is always due to an underlying disease process, which if treated successfully will cause the DIC to resolve on its own. In some cases, the treatment is easy and invariably successful, as in the removal of a dead fetus from the uterus. In other cases, such as a severely burned patient, only time can heal, and death may occur first.

(2) *Thrombotic thrombocytopenic purpura* (TTP). This disease's name is also decodable. *Thrombotic* means "clot-forming." The *thrombocytes* are the "clot cells," or platelets. *Penic* is from the Greek *penia*, "poverty," while *purpura* is the Latin word for "purple," and refers to the bruised-looking areas on the skin of someone who has suffered bleeding into the tissues immediately beneath. The full translation, then, is "a clot-forming disease, causing a low platelet count, producing bleeding." TTP is rare and its cause unknown, but it appears to be mediated by the immune system. Whatever the cause, there is damage to the internal lining of the small blood vessels, and clots form in the damaged areas. Although all this clotting uses up the patient's platelets, clotting proteins are not used up (in contrast to the situation in DIC). Nevertheless, since normal clotting cannot occur without platelets, the patient bleeds—hence "purpura." The hemolytic anemia that occurs as a result of red cells being disrupted by the clots may be very severe, requiring transfusion (while the anemia of DIC usually does not). A distinctive feature of TTP is that the effects of interrupted blood flow are especially apparent in the brain, and may result in a bizarre variety of neurological symptoms. Another target of damage is the kidney, as can be seen in DIC.

In the past, severe TTP had a very high mortality rate, about 90 percent. Nowadays, about 70 percent of cases can be cured or controlled by therapy. For reasons that are unclear, removal of the patient's plasma and replacement with normal plasma, called plasma exchange, is effective treatment. Modern plasma exchanges are done with an automated machine that continuously draws off a small quantity of the patient's whole blood, separates the cells from the plasma, returns the cells to the patient, and replaces the patient's plasma with donated plasma from volunteers. This continues until most of the patient's plasma has been replaced by normal donor plasma. Presumably there is some deleterious substance in the patient's plasma that incites the clotting and causes TTP, but no one yet knows what it is. Plasma exchange has to be done every day until the patient gets better, which is about nine days on the average. Most cases of TTP are acute, meaning that they occur once and either kill the patient or resolve with treatment, never to return; a few, however, are recurrent or chronic.

Other traumatic causes of hemolytic anemia

Passage through strands of clot in the small vessels is one way in which red cells become ruptured; other conditions can also produce sufficient physical stress on the red cells for hemolysis to occur. As may be expected in any system that develops over thousands of millennia, the circulatory system and the red cells work well together, hand-in-glove. The red cell has just enough tensile strength to withstand the pressures and turbulence forced upon it by the beating heart and the gantlet of valves that keep blood flowing in the proper direction. When humans meddle with the structure of the circulatory system, however, all bets are off. Even a structure as simple as a one-way heart valve cannot always be artificially reproduced with sufficient authenticity to avoid a degree of turbulence capable of destroying red cells. Therefore, some patients will experience a significant hemolytic anemia following surgery for replacement of a heart valve. Sometimes this anemia is so severe that the artificial valve itself has to be surgically replaced. Since this hemolysis occurs in the heart and large vessels leading from the heart, the condition is referred to as *macroangiopathic hemolytic anemia* (*macro-* meaning "large," the antonym of *micro-*, "small").

Physical activity that involves repetitive blows on the surfaces of the body can beat up red cells enough for clinical hemolytic anemia to develop. Because this condition was first noticed in soldiers after long forced marches, the name *march hemoglobinuria* has been applied. Nowadays, march hemoglobinuria is seen more commonly in long-distance runners than in infantry personnel, possibly because the latter have been equipped with better, more protective foot gear, and the former have become even more fanatic. March hemoglobinuria can also result from repeated blows to other body parts and has been observed in martial arts aficionados and players of conga and bongo drums.

Immunohemolytic anemia

We touched on the subject of autoimmune disease in the discussion of pernicious anemia in chapter 4. It turns out that autoantibodies attack not only intrinsic factor-producing cells in the stomach, but other tissues as well. When the body's immune system turns on its own red cells, hemolytic anemia can result. This brings us to the definition of immunohemolytic anemia: *that anemia which occurs as the result of destruction of red cells by antibodies.*

The normal function of antibodies is to defend the body against invaders. When a foreign substance (living or otherwise) composed of large complex molecules (like proteins and some carbohydrates) is introduced to the immune system, that system's response is to manufacture antibodies that attach to the surface of the foreign substance. When antibodies are attached to anything, the reticuloendothelial system recognizes the substance as an "enemy," and the macrophages and fixed phagocytes engulf that substance and destroy it. This works well as long as the antibody-producing cells know who the enemy is. In autoimmune diseases, some of the ability to tell friend from foe is lost, and antibodies arise that attack the host's own tissues. If that tissue is a red cell, antibodies coat those cells in the circulation, the RES recognizes them as the enemy, and the red cells are engulfed and destroyed. The result is clinical hemolytic anemia.

To make the diagnosis of immunohemolytic anemia, it is necessary to demonstrate that antibodies are attached to the surface of the anemic person's red cells. While they are large molecules by biological standards, antibodies are still far too

small to be seen with the microscope. Fortunately, the direct
Coombs test, which dates back to 1940, allows us to detect
antibody-coated red cells. In this test, we turn antibodies from
enemies back into friends by taking advantage of their property
of binding to other substances. First, the person's blood is
drawn, and the plasma is removed from the cells. The cells are
diluted and resuspended in an artificial liquid medium. Then,
the magical ingredient, antihuman red cell globulin (also called
"Coombs serum"), is added to the cell suspension. The Coombs
serum contains antibodies, originally derived from animals,
that specifically attach to human antibodies. (Since an antibody
is a large biological molecule itself, it is possible to make an
antibody against an antibody, in this case an animal antibody
against a human antibody.) If the anemic person's red cells are
coated with human antibodies, the animal-derived antibodies
in the Coombs serum will attach to them. Since the Coombs
serum antibodies have more than one attachment site for their
targets, they act as little bridges from one target molecule to
another. The result is the clumping together of the patient's
antibody-coated red cells, a phenomenon called agglutination.
Agglutination is readily visible with the naked eye, making the
direct Coombs test a simple procedure requiring no expensive
equipment (fig. 5.2).

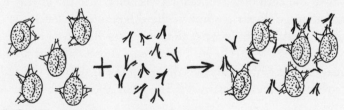

PATIENT'S ANTIBODY-
COATED RED CELLS

ANIMAL ANTIBODIES
THAT BIND TO HUMAN
ANTIBODIES

CELLS VISIBLY CLUMP UP

FIG. 5.2. The direct Coombs test

The most common immunohemolytic anemias are autoimmune diseases, but, as we shall see later, some immunohemolytic anemias are *alloimmune*; that is, they result from destruction of red cells by antibodies that an individual makes in normal response to stimulation by *another person's* red cells. First, we will deal with two autoimmune hemolytic anemias.

(1) *Warm autoimmune hemolytic anemia* (WAIHA). All antibodies are not created equal. Antibodies work better at lower than body temperature, which is not surprising, considering that the function of an antibody is to attach itself to something. Attachment is more difficult if the molecules of the attachment site are vibrating rapidly, and the higher the temperature, the faster the molecules vibrate. Accordingly, only the strongest of antibodies, called warm-reactive antibodies, are capable of binding to their targets at body temperature. The weaker cold antibodies are able to bind to their targets only at temperatures colder than normal body temperature. If a warm autoantibody is the cause of immunohemolytic anemia, the process of attachment can occur in any portion of the body, and the antibody-coated red cells are removed by the RES, causing hemolytic anemia.

Warm autoimmune hemolytic anemia can occur as an isolated disease, in which case it is termed *idiopathic WAIHA*. About half the cases, however, are manifestations of other diseases characterized by derangements or hyperstimulation of the immune system, including collagen-vascular diseases (e. g., lupus), infections, or lymphomas (cancers of the antibody-forming cells of the immune system). These anemias are called *secondary WAIHA*.

The treatment of WAIHA is aimed at controlling the rampaging immune response. The classic drugs employed in this effort are the *corticosteroids*, the most familiar being *prednisone*. Some corticosteroids are hormones naturally produced by the adrenal gland and are involved in a multitude of physiological station-keeping activities. Prednisone and its ilk are artificial analogues of the natural corticosteroid hormones. These drugs are used in the treatment of a variety of diseases characterized by overactivity of the immune system, from lupus to lymphoma. (Other antilymphoma drugs, such as cyclophosphamide and azathioprine, can be employed in cases where the less toxic corticosteroids do not work.)

About 80 percent of WAIHA cases respond favorably to corticosteroids. When these drugs fail, other treatments are available. One consists of huge doses of normal human antibodies given by IV injection, referred to as high-dose intravenous IgG ("IgG" stands for "immunoglobulin G," one of several chemical classes of antibodies in the circulation). Exactly how this treatment works is unknown, but it may involve the binding of IgG to the portions of the antibody-coated red cells recognized by the reticuloendothelial system, masking those autoantibodies from "view." If the RES does not recognize the red cells as being antibody-coated, then it has no reason to remove them from the circulation and destroy them.

For cases of WAIHA that do not respond to drugs of any kind, the anemic person's spleen may be surgically removed. This procedure, *splenectomy*, gets rid of the most persnickety organ of the RES. The other RES organs (bone marrow and liver) have a more live-and-let-live philosophy concerning antibody-coated red cells, so removal of the spleen may result in increased red cell survival in WAIHA.

(2) *Cold agglutinin disease* (CAD). Some autoantibodies are weaker than those that cause warm autoimmune hemolytic anemia and can coat red cells only at temperatures below normal core body temperature (98.6 degrees Fahrenheit, or 37 degrees Celsius). It would seem logical that these cold agglutinins, as they are termed, would never cause any trouble, since the body maintains a constant temperature (except in fever, when the temperature is even higher). In fact, the extremities of the body do not maintain as high a temperature as that found in the core. Extremity temperature is even more variable for those who live in a cold environment.

Interestingly, all normal individuals have cold agglutinins floating around in their plasma (the function is unknown), and these do not cause any problems. In cases of cold agglutinin disease, however, the concentration of cold agglutinins rises manyfold, to as much as 100,000 times normal. In such enormous amounts, cold agglutinins not only coat red cells but also cause them to clump together and block up small blood vessels. Since the cold agglutinins react only at lower temperatures, this plugging up of vessels occurs in the extremities and is most pronounced in cold environments. The clinical symptoms, in addition to those of hemolytic anemia, include pain and numbness in the fingers, toes, nose, cheeks, and ears, where body temperature is the lowest. The affected areas become starved for oxygen, and the hemoglobin in the vessels turns purple. The overlying skin loses the normal pink appearance lent by fully oxygenated hemoglobin and takes on the dusky blue color of the deoxygenated hemoglobin, a clinical sign referred to as *cyanosis*. In some cases the oxygen starvation is so severe there is actual death of tissue, or *necrosis*, resulting in loss of fingers and toes.

Cold agglutinin disease may be idiopathic, but more often it results from one of several primary causes, including lymphomas and certain infections. Cases of CAD that accompany infectious mononucleosis and a common form of pneumonia, namely that caused by the bacterium *Mycoplasma hominis*, typically resolve along with the primary infection.

Chronic cases of CAD are treated first by simple common-sense means, such as the wearing of gloves and other warm clothing. Some people elect to deal with their problem by moving to a warmer climate. Expensive heated environmental suits are available for those who choose to stay in cold climates. Plasma exchange, mentioned above in the discussion of thrombotic thrombocytopenic purpura, will readily remove the cold agglutinins, but the deranged immune system just replaces them. Unfortunately, corticosteroids and splenectomy, so useful in WAIHA, are ineffective in cold agglutinin disease.

The next two immunohemolytic anemias are alloimmune, that is, they result from antibodies made by an individual against another person's red cells:

(1) *Hemolytic transfusion reaction* is a hemolytic anemia that occurs when the normal antibodies of a transfusion recipient coat and destroy red cells transfused from a donor. Fortunately, because modern blood banking is fanatic in its observation of safety procedures, hemolytic transfusion reactions are extremely rare.

(2) *Hemolytic disease of the newborn* (HDN). The pregnant woman provides her fetus with oxygen and nutrients through an interface organ called the placenta. The function of the placenta is to allow nutrient molecules and oxygen to pass from the mother's circulation into that of the fetus, and to allow carbon dioxide and waste molecules to pass from fetus to mother. Ideally, the circulations of the mother and fetus are kept separate from each other. In reality, the placenta is not perfect in this regard, and some minor amount of blood usually escapes, passing from the fetus into the mother and vice versa. Since the genetic makeup of the fetus is divided roughly half-and-half between its mother and father, the fetus is "half different" from its mother. In some cases the red cells of the fetus have surface molecules, called red cell antigens, programmed by the father's genes, that would be recognized as foreign by the mother's immune system. If exposed to these foreign antigens, the mother's immune system would manufacture antibodies against them. Such antibodies may be able to cross the placental barrier and destroy the red cells of the fetus as it rests unsuspectingly in its warm, watery environment. The result is hemolytic anemia arising even before birth. This anemia, if severe, causes such a pronounced stimulation of the fetus's marrow in compensatory response that fully nucleated, immature red cells (erythroblasts) stream out into the bloodstream in huge numbers. This phenomenon provides the classical name for the severe, potentially fatal alloimmune hemolytic anemia of the fetus and newborn: *erythroblastosis fetalis*.

Hemolytic disease of the newborn is more than just an anemia. Although the anemia itself can be quite serious, there is a second threat to the baby, and that is the *toxic effect of bilirubin*. Jaundice in newborns occurs not only because of hemolysis, but also because the neonatal liver is just not up to speed and cannot handle even a normal amount of red cell removal. This is why even perfectly normal newborns can become slightly jaundiced for a few days. Add hemolysis to that picture, and the jaundice can become severe. In the adult, a high level of bilirubin by itself causes no clinical problems. The worst it can do is give the skin and mucous membranes an aesthetically unappealing cast. Bilirubin is normally toxic to the brain, but, in the adult, the so-called blood-brain barrier is so well developed that bilirubin in the plasma cannot get into the brain to harm it. In newborn babies, the blood-brain barrier is not fully developed, so bilirubin freely crosses from plasma into the brain, causing permanent neurological damage. This complication of HDN is called *kernicterus* ("icterus" meaning "jaundice," and "kern-" referring to the anatomic parts of the brain that are damaged).

A detailed discussion of HDN is beyond the scope of this book, but it is worth noting that simple, routine prenatal care can prevent the vast majority of potential cases. This is one of numerous reasons why it is extremely important for any woman to seek qualified medical care as soon as she has reason to believe she is pregnant.

Hypersplenism

As we have seen, the spleen is one of the major sites of red cell destruction, both in the normal state and in immunohemolytic anemia. In either case, the spleen is simply doing its jobs, those being the removal and disassembly of red cells at the end of their life span and the removal of any objects (good or bad) that are coated with antibodies. Since Murphy's Law applies to virtually every organ of the body, it is not surprising that even the spleen can malfunction. The normal spleen is not supposed to destroy normal (nonantibody-coated) red cells until they are old. In cases where the spleen is enlarged (a condition called *splenomegaly*), red cells are held in the organ longer than usual while they meander around the splenic sinusoids finding their way out. The temptation is too much for the fixed phagocytes and macrophages, which, when confronted with red cells that tarry too long, engulf and destroy them. The result is hemolytic anemia, and the condition is termed *hypersplenism*.

Any disease that causes the spleen to be enlarged can cause hypersplenism. Several examples are:

(1) *Cirrhosis of the liver*. Cirrhosis is a chronic, irreversible destructive condition that progressively causes the liver to become scarred, or fibrotic. As the scar tissue forms, it becomes more and more difficult for blood entering the liver to get through it and back to the heart. The major vein that drains into the liver is the portal vein, the function of which is to convey nutrients from the digestive tract straight to the liver, where so much reassembly of nutrients into proteins and carbohydrates occurs. In cirrhosis, the fibrotic liver interferes with the portal vein circulation, causing back pressure on the vein. This condition is called portal hypertension. Portal hypertension causes a host of health problems, but the one that concerns us here derives from the fact that one of the major tributaries of the portal vein is the splenic vein, the main vein that drains the spleen. The elevated pressure in the portal vein is reflected back into the spleen, causing it to gradually blow up like a balloon; hypersplenism is one upshot.

(2) *Infections*. Some infections, such as typhoid fever, infectious mononucleosis, malaria, and kala-azar (a parasitic infection of tropical regions) can cause splenomegaly, leading to hypersplenism.

(3) *Lymphomas*. These or other hematologic malignancies can involve the spleen. The cancer cells proliferate there, causing the whole organ to enlarge. Hypersplenism can result.

The treatment of hypersplenism boils down to either treating the primary disease that caused the splenomegaly in the first place, or, failing that, surgically removing the spleen. Splenectomy is a fairly safe procedure in otherwise healthy individuals, but in patients with debilitating diseases (such as cirrhosis and cancer), the postoperative mortality from the surgery is relatively high (10 percent or more). Moreover, the spleen is not an unessential organ, since it plays a major role in fighting off infections by certain bacteria. The decision to remove the spleen, therefore, should not be taken lightly.

OTHER HEMOLYTIC ANEMIAS

An important category of hemolytic anemias is composed of those that result from a hereditary, genetic defect. The defect may be in the structure of hemoglobin (hemoglobinopathies), the mechanism determining the rate at which hemoglobin is synthesized (thalassemias), the structure of the red cell membrane (hereditary spherocytosis), and the enzymes that help maintain a safe environment for hemoglobin in the cell (glucose-6-phosphate dehydrogenase deficiency). These hemolytic anemias will be discussed along with other hereditary anemias in chapter 6.

IN SUMMARY

Hemolytic anemias are those caused by a shortened red cell life span. They are classified as normocytic, normochromic anemias. The diagnosis of hemolytic anemia is made by demonstrating a normal marrow response to the anemia, best measured by the reticulocyte count. Other tests, such as serum bilirubin, serum haptoglobin, urine urobilinogen, urine hemoglobin, and examination of the blood smear may also be helpful. The characteristic laboratory findings in a generic case of hemolytic anemia are given in the table below:

Test	Expected Result
hemoglobin	low
MCV	normal*
MCHC	normal
serum total bilirubin	mildly elevated
serum direct bilirubin	normal
serum indirect bilirubin	mildly elevated
serum haptoglobin	low or absent
urine urobilinogen	elevated

*In some very severe hemolytic anemias with very high reticulocyte counts, the MCV may be slightly elevated, since reticulocytes are slightly larger than normal red cells.

Hemolysis may occur as a result of physical trauma to red cells (DIC, TTP, march hemoglobinuria), destruction of antibody-coated red cells by the RES (WAIHA, cold agglutinin disease, hemolytic transfusion reactions, hemolytic disease of the newborn), and any condition that results in an enlarged spleen (hypersplenism). The treatment and prognosis of hemolytic anemia depend on the underlying cause.

6. Inherited Anemias

Even red blood cells may fall victim to Old Testament justice, with the hematologic woes of the parents being inflicted on succeeding generations of their issue. In some cases (sickle cell disease, for instance), the method behind evolution's madness can be fathomed, but there seems to be no explanation for the existence of most of these diseases beyond some multigenerational version of Murphy's Law. Most of the anemias discussed in this chapter are cytometrically classified as normocytic, normochromic (normal MCV and MCHC), and most are hemolytic anemias (the exceptions being thalassemia and hemoglobin E disease, which are microcytic, hypochromic). If you have not read chapter 5, doing so would help you become familiar with hemolytic anemia in general.

HEMOGLOBINOPATHIES

Briefly defined, a hemoglobinopathy is *any condition characterized by an abnormal structure of the globin chain of hemoglobin*. Note that the word "anemia" does not enter into the definition. This is because not all hemoglobinopathies lead to anemia. Before we discuss the ones that do, we will cover hemoglobin biochemistry in a little more depth.

As we saw in chapter 1, hemoglobin is composed of a protein component called globin and four molecules of heme. Globin actually consists of four long chains of amino acids, each of which is called a *subunit*. The normal adult hemoglobin molecule consists of two copies each of two subunits, called *alpha* and *beta*. Since a total of four subunits combine to make the globin molecule, that molecule is referred to as a *tetramer* (from Greek roots *tetra-*, "four" and *-mer*, "part"). Each subunit is nothing more than a long sequence of amino acids programmed according to a sequence of nucleotides on a DNA molecule. This nucleotide sequence is called a gene. For globin, there is one gene for the construction of alpha subunits and one gene for beta subunits. The alpha and beta genes are inherited independently from each other; in fact, these genes are on different chromosomes.

When any protein molecule, including a globin subunit, is constructed by translation from a gene template, the long chain of amino acids does not stay all strung out waving randomly like a long rope floating in a lake. Rather, each long chain folds up into a blob with a very specific shape, which is dictated by the interactions among the various different amino acids on the chain. There is a total of 20 different amino acids in human proteins, each of which has a different size, shape, and electric charge from those of the others. Some attract each other, some repel. The resulting complete protein molecule has a defined three-dimensional shape, which is what determines its function. In the case of globin, each subunit has to be properly shaped to (1) hold on to the other three subunits with just enough strength so that they can hinge on each other to properly adjust oxygen-binding ability as the hemoglobin molecule loads up with oxygen, and (2) hold on to heme with just the right amount of force so that oxygen can be transported but then given up to the tissues.

The hemoglobin molecule is built so delicately that it is simply a disaster waiting to happen. A variety of misfortunes can befall this vital molecule, which explains why the red cell expends nearly all its meager energy supply keeping the hemoglobin molecule safe and happy. If a mutation (an accidental alteration of the gene nucleotide sequence) occurs in the DNA that determines the structure of a globin subunit, there may be subtle or not-so-subtle changes in the three-dimensional structure of hemoglobin. Like the effect of red kryptonite on Superman, the result of a globin structural mutation is pretty much unpredictable. Possible effects of such a mutation are:

(1) *No observable effect.* This is in fact the usual result of a random mutation. There are "silent" areas of the amino acid sequence of globin that do not affect its ultimate biochemical function. For this reason, most hemoglobinopathies are never clinically detected, and are simply fodder for the research scientist.

(2) *Altered hemoglobin-oxygen affinity.* Some mutations result in a strengthening or weakening of the bond between hemoglobin and oxygen. If the bond is too tight, oxygen will not be delivered as well to the tissues. Oxygen starvation at the tissue level sends a signal to the marrow to make more red cells. This results in a red cell count, hematocrit, and hemoglobin level that is *too high.* This condition is called *polycythemia*, which is the opposite of anemia (there are other, more common causes of polycythemia, but they are beyond the scope of this book).

If the affinity between hemoglobin and oxygen is too low, then oxygen is too readily released from hemoglobin and is not transported to the tissues. The presence of the purple deoxygenated hemoglobin in the circulation gives the patient a dusky blue complexion, expressed by the clinical term cyanosis (again, there are other more common, nonhematological causes of cyanosis, which are not discussed here).

(3) *Physical destabilization of hemoglobin.* Most proteins in biological systems are suspended in their watery medium like salt dissolved in water. The individual protein molecules are free to move over each other in any direction, so that the medium in which they are suspended behaves like a liquid and is easily deformable. This physical state of proteins is called the sol state. A familiar example of the sol state is the white of an uncooked egg. Hemoglobin must stay in the sol state to allow the red cells to be deformed sufficiently to squeeze through the tiny capillaries of the circulation. Under sufficient chemical or thermal stress, any sol-state protein can be transformed to the gel state, which is physically more like a rubbery solid. The white of a hard-boiled egg is an example of the gel state. If

hemoglobin is sufficiently stressed, or because of its abnormal structure is rendered unusually susceptible to stress, then it, too, can transform into the gel state. Cells containing gelled hemoglobin cannot make it through the circulation, because the ever-vigilant reticuloendothelial system senses those cells as abnormal and destroys them, causing a hemolytic anemia. Some mutations yield an abnormal structure that just causes the hemoglobin to gel out into spherical blobs, which can be seen under the microscope when certain special stains are used. These blobs are called *Heinz bodies*. At least one other globin mutation produces rectangular crystals of gelled hemoglobin. This is called *hemoglobin C*. The most notorious type of unstable hemoglobin is one that causes hemoglobin to form up into long skeins of protein that grossly deform the red cells into bizarre, elongated, double-pointed monstrosities that are not only destroyed by the RES, but jam up together and interfere with the circulation throughout the body. These mutant hemoglobins are collectively called *sickling hemoglobins*, and the most infamous of these by far is *hemoglobin S*, the cause of *sickle cell anemia*.

Over 400 hemoglobinopathies have been described by indefatigable biochemists over the decades, but it is necessary to discuss only three here—hemoglobin S, hemoglobin C, and hemoglobin E. Each of these mutations involves only one error in its beta globin chain—the replacement of the correct amino acid by an incorrect one in a specific position on the chain. We all inherit any given gene in pairs, one from the mother and one from the father (except for genes on the X and Y chromosomes, but they are of no concern in relation to globin genes). In the cases of hemoglobins S, C, and E, inheritance of the abnormal gene from only one parent causes little or no clinical abnormality, so this condition is called a hemoglobin S, C, or E *trait*. If however, you inherit one copy of the abnormal gene from each parent, so that you get a double dose, you are said to have hemoglobin S, C, or E *disease*. In the case of trait, the normal gene makes enough hemoglobin A to outweigh the effects of the abnormal hemoglobin made by the mutated gene.

In the case of disease, however, no hemoglobin A is made, so the only hemoglobin synthesized is the abnormal one.

An important feature of hemoglobins S, C, and E is that they contain beta chain mutations. Beta chains are not normally synthesized in significant amounts until the age of six months. Before that time, the predominant hemoglobin is composed of two alpha chains and two *gamma* chains. This is called *hemoglobin F* ("F" stands for "fetal"). Because hemoglobin A, with its beta chains, does not take over until age six months (the same is true of hemoglobins S, C, and E with their mutated beta chains), these diseases are not clinically manifest until then.

SICKLE CELL DISEASE (HEMOGLOBIN S DISEASE)

Among inherited anemias, sickle cell disease is the most prominent, not only because of its prevalence in the United States but also because of the level of misery and debility it causes. (For a more detailed discussion of this disease than can be given here, see another title in this series, *Understanding Sickle Cell Disease* by Miriam Bloom.)

Although this is thought of as a "black disease," the hemoglobin S gene has been detected in white populations, especially those of Mediterranean ancestry. Still, in the U.S. the disease is almost always observed in African Americans and others of sub-Saharan African origin. The prevalence of the gene in the U.S. is about 9 percent, but some population enclaves in Africa have a much higher incidence, as high as 45 percent. Despite the high prevalence of the gene in the U.S., only 0.14 percent of blacks in this counry have actual sickle cell disease. The rest of the gene carriers have sickle cell trait and are not sick.

The sickle cell mutation is one for which we understand the evolutionary "reason." Individuals with sickle cell trait are particularly resistant to a certain form of malaria called falciparum malaria. This is a rather nasty disease, and it is much more important as a cause of death in tropical regions than is sickle cell disease. It is not surprising then that the sickle cell gene has propagated so successfully in a subset of humanity whose origins lie in the tropics. (Another major disease for which we understand the "reason" is cystic fibrosis; the gene confers resistance to another dreaded infectious disease, cholera.)

Like all beta chain mutations, sickle cell anemia is not apparent until the age of six months, when the beta chain-bearing hemoglobin takes over the lion's share of the work from hemoglobin F. The clinical manifestations are those of a severe hemolytic anemia, with all its signs and symptoms. In addition, because of the tendency for sickled cells to glom up and block the microcirculation, many painful and destructive complications occur:

(1) *Dactylitis* is painful swelling of the fingers and toes caused by loss of circulation to the small bones in those areas. This is often the first sign of sickle cell anemia in a baby.

(2) *Infarctive crisis*, also called "painful crisis," often occurs when the body is under stress, as from an acute infection. Any organ can be affected by the oxygen starvation wrought by snarled plugs of sickled red cells. Loss of tissue viability downstream from any plugged blood vessel is called an infarction, and it not only causes excruciating pain, but can also produce enough tissue death to interfere with organ function. If this happens to the heart, the result may be a myocardial infarction, or heart attack, a potentially fatal condition that occurs in people with sickle cell at a much younger age than it does in the non-sickle cell population. One organ that is almost invariably lost by the person's teen years is the spleen. Repetitive infarctions of splenic tissue during childhood cause the spleen to scar down to a useless nubbin. This process is called autosplenectomy.

(3) *Leg ulcers* are caused by loss of circulation to the lower extremities. Some people with sickle cell who are otherwise tolerating their disease well are plagued by these nonhealing sores, occurring most often just above the ankle.

(4) *Infections* represent the most common immediate cause of death among people with sickle cell. This is partially due to the loss of spleen function, but other poorly understood factors may also play some role.

(5) *Priapism* (named after the Greek fertility god Priapus, typically represented with an erect phallus) is a painful, sustained erection of the penis caused by obstruction of the blood vessels that drain this organ. In a normal sexual response, these vessels constrict in response to neural stimulation by the brain, causing blood to fill up the cavernous spaces in the penis and resulting in an erection. After orgasm or subsidence of sexual stimulation, these vessels open up to let the blood out. In sickle cell anemia, these vessels are plugged up by sickled cells, so blood cannot escape normally. Most of these attacks resolve on their own, but occasionally an attack that lasts over 24 hours can cause the cavernous spaces to become filled with scar tissue, and the person then suffers impotence.

Better management of sickle cell anemia has been developing over the past few decades. At one time, the only treatment that could be offered was pain medication and blood transfusions. Recent advances in treatment have focused on manipulating the bone marrow into producing hemoglobin F. Although fetal hemoglobin is best adapted for intrauterine life before birth, it can serve quite well as an oxygen carrier even in the adult, and it is certainly not as deleterious to the body as hemoglobin S. Even though a normal adult produces little or no hemoglobin F, every red cell precursor silently harbors the gamma chain gene that would make the production of this hemoglobin possible. The gene is simply switched off after early infancy. The current drug of choice for turning the gamma gene back on is hydroxyurea, better known for its longtime use in treatment of certain cancers. This drug blocks methyl group transfer (the reaction that uses folate, as discussed in chapter 4) and thus inhibits DNA synthesis, but apparently the blockage of this vital reaction causes silent genes to be reactivated. As expected, hydroxyurea produces megaloblastic anemia as a side effect, but its derepression of the gamma chain gene makes up for its undesirable properties. A less toxic drug that also stimulates the production of hemoglobin F is butyrate, a simple organic acid familiar to many as the chemical that gives rancid butter its characteristic unpleasant odor.

The great hope for people with sickle cell is the promise of genetic engineering, by which normal beta genes would be introduced into their own erythroblasts. Research is very active in this area. In the meantime, the few attempts at bone marrow transplantation have resulted in some cures. The problems with this include a significant rate of short-term mortality (about 20 percent) and the availability of a suitable donor (usually a sibling).

HEMOGLOBIN C DISEASE

Hemoglobin C is similar to hemoglobin S in several ways. First, it is seen almost entirely in black people of African origin (it is even more exclusively confined to blacks than hemoglobin S is). Second, it results from an amino acid substitution at exactly the same position as the one for hemoglobin S. Finally, the instability of hemoglobin C produces an organized structure in the red cell. However, this structure is a rectangular, blunt-ended crystal, rather than the long, skinny, pointed structure formed by destabilized hemoglobin S. That difference is enough to make the clinical disease caused by hemoglobin C quite different from sickle cell disease.

Hemoglobin C disease is a simple hemolytic anemia, with no observable effects related to any blood vessel obstruction. Apparently, crystallized hemoglobin C cells can still flow pretty well, unlike sickle cells. The RES is not fooled however, and the nonconformist crystallized cells are removed from the circulation with alacrity. The prevalence of hemoglobin C trait in African Americans is about 2.4 percent, with hemoglobin C disease being observed in about 0.02 percent. In Africa, the prevalence of the trait can be as high as 26 percent. Although less frequent than hemoglobin S, hemoglobin C is still more common than any other hemoglobinopathy in the U.S., and is third behind hemoglobin S and hemoglobin E worldwide.

The anemia of hemoglobin C is typically mild and usually does not require any treatment. It is important for the physician to recognize this condition, though, to prevent unnecessary treatment resulting from erroneous diagnoses.

HEMOGLOBIN E DISEASE

As a result of the wave of migration from Southeast Asia beginning in the 1970s, hemoglobin E is no longer a rarity in medical practice in the U.S. The second most common hemoglobinopathy in the world (after sickle cell disease), this mutation is characterized by a single amino acid substitution, at a position on the beta chain different from the one in hemoglobins S and C. Hemoglobin E is most common in Thailand and Burma, where prevalence of trait is between 10 percent and 20 percent of the population. In hemoglobin E disease, the abnormal hemoglobin does not physically destabilize, as with hemoglobins S and C. Instead, the mutation causes the formation of unstable RNA, the intermediary between the DNA gene and the finished globin beta protein chain. The result is a decreased level of RNA, resulting in a reduced rate of hemoglobin production. The resulting red cells are small (low MCV) and pale (low MCHC) because of their lack of hemoglobin. Hemoglobin E disease, then, is manifested as a microcytic, hypochromic anemia. The anemia is mild and requires no treatment, but, since it can masquerade as iron deficiency, it is commonly misdiagnosed as such. Accordingly, it is important for the doctor to recognize that a mild microcytic anemia in an individual of Southeast Asian heritage may be due to this hemoglobinopathy.

THALASSEMIA

Hemoglobin E disease is a hemoglobinopathy in which a structural defect in a globin chain gene causes a decreased rate of synthesis of the chain, resulting in retarded synthesis of hemoglobin. There are many other inherited conditions that are characterized by decreased rate of hemoglobin synthesis *without* a defect in the amino acid structure of a globin chain. These are called *thalassemias*. The term is taken from the ancient Greek word *thalassa*, meaning sea, because the first descriptions of serious forms of this disease involved people of Mediterranean heritage. As other less serious, even silent, forms of thalassemia were discovered, it became apparent that the condition was not limited to that geographic area. In fact, the various thalassemia genes are distributed among populations that arose from a broad, world-encircling tropical belt including the Mediterranean, sub-Saharan Africa, the Middle East, the Indian subcontinent, Southeast Asia, and the East Indies (Native American populations are remarkably free of thalassemia and hemoglobinopathy genes).

A working definition of thalassemia is *an inherited condition in which there is decreased synthesis of a globin chain that is structurally normal* (cf. hemoglobinopathies, in which a globin chain has an abnormal structure). Thalassemias represent an extraordinarily diverse group of conditions, and entire volumes have been written on just the genetics of this disease. Since the abnormality may affect the alpha or the beta chain (or sometimes both), there are two major categories of thalassemia, *alpha-thalassemia* and *beta-thalassemia*. In each of these categories, there is a variety of mutations that result in a wide spectrum of reduced globin synthesis. Some conditions cause complete cessation of synthesis, while others cause only a mild decrease.

Things get even more complicated when one considers that each individual inherits two corresponding globin chain genes (one from each parent), and the abnormalities conveyed by the various genes have an additive effect. For instance, one person (call him "Bill") who has inherited two copies of a beta-thal gene coding for only a mild decrease in beta synthesis may have the same mild condition as another person ("Sally") who inherited only one copy of a gene that conveys a more severe abnormality. Accordingly, two individuals who share the same *phenotype* (referring to the apparent expression of the gene) have different *genotypes* (referring to the actual structure of the gene itself). To complicate things further, consider the possibility that Bill and Sally will meet in the waiting room at the hematologist's office, fall in love, and proceed to raise a family. All of their children will inherit one of Bill's abnormal genes for mild beta-thal. Half of them will inherit Sally's gene for severe beta-thal. Those who do will get a double dose of a beta-thalassemia gene, one of which is a severe variant. These children may then suffer from a moderately severe form of the disease that requires lifelong clinical intervention.

The challenge of understanding thalassemia can be met by simplifying the bewildering cacophony of minutiae into a few distilled rules. We will look first at alpha-thalassemia, which, although extremely common, is rarely a clinical problem in the U.S., and then beta-thalassemia, which is less common but clinically more significant.

Alpha-thalassemia

In alpha thalassemia, insufficient amounts of alpha globin chains are synthesized. There are two abnormal genes for this condition, called alpha-thal-1 and alpha-thal-2. The alpha-thal-1 gene (which is actually a combination of two genes in a row, both of which are defective) allows the synthesis of no alpha chains, while the alpha-thal-2 gene (also composed of two genes, only one of which is defective) allows the synthesis of some alpha chains, but not a normal amount.

Beta-thalassemia

Beta-thalassemias are actually more complicated than alpha-thalassemias, since there are about 100 different mutations affecting beta chain synthesis in various world populations, each of which causes different levels of severity. These genes tend to center in certain ethnic/racial groups, namely Mediterranean peoples, Asian Indians, African blacks, Chinese, and Southeast Asians. Although the genetics of this disease is a formidable subject, all cases of beta-thal can be classified into one of three groups based on the clinical severity of the disease: thalassemia minor, thalassemia major, and thalassemia intermedia.

Thalassemia minor is the mildest form. It is seen in those who have inherited one normal beta chain gene and one abnormal one. Affected individuals have no anemia or a mild, asymptomatic anemia (hemoglobin levels between 10 and 12 grams per deciliter) requiring no treatment. The characteristic hematological finding is marked microcytosis (low MCV) and a *high* RBC count. In other words, the person with thal minor has *lots of little red cells*. A correct diagnosis is important, because thal minor can be mistaken for iron deficiency, and the person would be subjected to iron therapy unnecessarily. It is also important for the affected individual to know about the situation, because marriage to another person with thal minor could yield children with thal major, which is a serious condition.

Thalassemia major is the dreaded disease first described in children of Mediterranean origin by Dr. Thomas Cooley (the disease is also known as Cooley's anemia). This disease is seen in people who have inherited one mutated beta chain gene from each parent. Thal major has so many ramifications throughout the body that to learn the pathophysiology of this disease is to learn a lot about hematology in general. It is therefore useful to consider thalassemia major in depth.

Up to this point, we have thought of thalassemia as a sort of faux iron deficiency anemia that results in decreased hemoglobin synthesis, causing a microcytic, hypochromic anemia. In fact, the situation is much worse than that. While iron deficiency simply causes hemoglobin to be produced in insufficient amounts, thalassemia not only does that but also causes an imbalance between the number of globin chains that make up the hemoglobin molecule. In the case of beta-thal, the synthesis of beta chains is retarded, but alpha chains are synthesized at a normal rate. The extra alpha chains don't just sit around doing nothing. Since they are constructed with the intent of forming protein tetramers (four-subunit proteins), when they find insufficient numbers of beta chains to bind with, they simply bind with themselves. The resultant protein is called an alpha-tetramer. These proteins are extremely unstable and actually kill the red cells in which they accumulate. Some of the red cells that fall victim to alpha-tetramers are already out in the peripheral circulation, so the result is some degree of hemolytic anemia. The tetramers are so toxic that most of the red cells are killed while still in the marrow. The marrow fills up and overflows with dying erythroblasts, and those that have not yet died off respond to the anemia by dividing even more rapidly and becoming more numerous. This is *ineffective erythropoiesis* (a term we are familiar with from the discussion of megaloblastic anemias in chapter 4). As the mass of erythroblasts increases, the marrow is not voluminous enough to hold all this tissue. Colonies of red cell precursors seed out into other organs throughout the body and form large masses of red-cell-forming tissues, a phenomenon called *extramedullary hematopoiesis*. This is especially apparent in the RES, so one of the prominent physical findings in thal major is enlargement of the spleen and liver, or *hepatosplenomegaly*. The spleen may become so enlarged that hypersplenism results (see chapter 5), contributing further to the hemolytic anemia. To add insult to injury, the rapid turnover in the wildly dividing red cell precursors causes such a strain on the machinery of DNA synthesis that folate is used up faster than it can be replaced from the diet. This causes a secondary megaloblastic state, making the anemia worse.

To summarize, the severe anemia in beta-thalassemia major is caused by an additive combination of all the following factors:

   a. Decreased hemoglobin production secondary to decreased synthesis of beta chains.

   b. Hemolysis caused by the toxic effects of alpha-tetramers.

c. Ineffective erythropoiesis, again due to alpha-tetramers.
d. Hypersplenism due to extramedullary hematopoiesis.
e. Megaloblastic anemia, because folate becomes depleted through the energetic production of doomed red cell precursors.

Beta-thal major is a disease that begins around the age of six months as hemoglobin F disappears (remember that mutations affecting beta chains are masked at birth because fetal hemoglobin has perfectly normal gamma chains in their place). The anemia that develops is profound, with hemoglobin levels in the range of 2 to 7 grams per deciliter (normal range for an adult male is 14–18). In growing youngsters, the bones themselves form around the markedly expanded marrow, causing deformities of the face and skull. One bone that is especially inclined to expand disproportionately to its neighbors is the upper jaw, or maxilla, which then grossly overhangs the lower jaw to give an appearance called chipmunk facies (*facies*, the Latin word for "face," is the medical term used to describe facial shapes in various conditions). The frontal bones of the skull also enlarge and produce dome-shaped protuberances, referred to as frontal bossing. The classic X-ray appearance of the thickened skull in thal major has been dubbed the "hair on end appearance."

Children with thalassemia major suffer severe growth retardation and may never progress to sexual maturity. This is at least partially due to the tremendous nutritional drain impressed on the victim by the runaway bone marrow and extramedullary hematopoietic tissues.

Ironically, the treatment for thalassemia major is the cause of death for these children. As the anemia worsens in infancy, it is necessary to give repeated blood transfusions. The problem is that the child's body does not have the necessary machinery to dispose of the tremendous amount of iron that each transfusion brings with it. The surplus iron quickly fills up the RES and then starts being deposited in other tissues. Like other trace metals, iron is toxic in excessive amounts; the heart, liver, and pancreas are especially susceptible to its destructive effects. In the heart, destruction of muscle cells causes congestive heart failure. In the liver, the result is cirrhosis. Iron deposits cause the pancreas to lose the ability to secrete pancreatic digestive enzymes, resulting in malabsorption, which worsens the patient's nutritional status. The term for the disease caused by toxic accumulations of iron is hemochromatosis (although most cases of hemochromatosis are due to other, nonhematological causes).

Fortunately, there is treatment for transfusion-induced hemochromatosis called *chelation therapy* (this should not be confused with the chelation therapy advocated by various "alternative medicine" proponents for a wide variety of common diseases unrelated to metal toxicity; no one has ever shown that this form of chelation works). The word "chelation" comes from the Greek word for "claw." Drugs used for this purpose react with the target metal atoms by picking them up between pincer-like extensions of the drug's molecular structure. The chelator, with the metal atom in tow, is then eliminated in the urine. The most commonly used chelator is deferoxamine (marketed under the trade name Desferal), which must be given by injection, either intravenously or subcutaneously (under the skin). Despite chelation's benefits, iron and its toxic effects still accumulate, albeit at a slower pace, and the person with thalassemia major does not enjoy a normal life expectancy. Currently, research is under way for the development of L1, a chelating drug that can be given by mouth. This should give some measure of relief to those children who have to endure the pain of the nine- to twelve-hour daily subcutaneously pumped injections of deferoxamine.

Bone marrow transplantation has been done in a few hundred infants with thal major, and results have been good. There is something of a Catch-22 involved in the decision to perform a transplant. For the transplant to have the best opportunity of surviving and not causing complications, the procedure has to be done early in life. The problem is that beta-thalassemia exhibits such a wide spectrum of severity that it is impossible to predict how severely affected a given person might be. Accordingly, a number of transplants might be done on babies who would never need them. Moreover, transplantation is not harmless, carrying with it a significant incidence of mortality (the discussion of aplastic anemia in chapter 7 contains more detail about bone marrow transplantation).

A hot topic of research in this area is the use of umbilical cord blood as a source of donor tissue. Blood left in the cord that is not needed by the newborn baby contains the primitive precursor cells that are capable of repopulating a recipient's marrow. Umbilical cord blood transplantation may not involve as big a risk to the recipient as donated marrow from an older individual. Moreover, it is possible that unmatched, unrelated donors can be employed. This is an exciting line of inquiry that will continue to develop over the next few years. Of course, as with all inherited diseases, the great hope lies in gene therapy, but at present this is just a dream.

Thalassemia intermedia occurs in individuals who have inherited a double dose of genes for the milder forms of thalassemia or a gene for a severe form and one normal gene. These patients naturally maintain a hemoglobin level of between 7 and 10 grams per deciliter. This level is well tolerated, and such individuals suffer few health problems as a result. Transfusion is usually not required, so that iron toxicity is not a problem.

G6PD DEFICIENCY

As we have seen, the duty of the red cell is to give aid and comfort to hemoglobin. This is a demanding job, for hemoglobin is not only a fragile protein incapable of existing outside the cell, but it is also charged with transporting a potentially deadly cargo, oxygen molecules. Oxygen is probably one of the most dangerous substances in the biological world. It is chemically highly reactive and can cause the destruction of a host of biological molecules. It is likely that the early living world existed without free atmospheric oxygen for billions of years. The primitive organisms that inhabited such a world drew meager amounts of energy from minerals and simple organic molecules in their surroundings. Evolution then took a giant step with photosynthesis, through which primitive one-celled plants could capture energy from sunlight. With time, plants developed into increasingly complex, more massive organisms. As the mass of plants expanded, the waste product of photosynthesis, free oxygen, began to fill the atmosphere. Evolution accommodated the energy lust of ever more mobile organisms, allowing animal life as we know it to develop.

Oxygen's high reactivity is the reason that this gas, which gives life, can also destroy it. The burning of wood, paper, or petroleum is nothing more than an uncontrolled version of the same chemical reaction by which sugars are metabolized in the body. Oxygen in the red cells can fall prey to toxic chemicals that are capable of donating electrons one at a time. These one-electron oxygen molecules represent a class of highly reactive substances called *free radicals*. The one-electron oxygen free radical eventually is converted to hydrogen peroxide, which itself breaks down into other free radicals capable of doing such damage to hemoglobin and other red cell structures that the cell is destroyed, resulting in hemolytic anemia. The chemicals that initiate this mayhem include the antimalaria drug primaquine, the antileprosy drug dapsone, the class of commonly prescribed antimicrobial drugs called sulfonamides, including sulfamethoxazole (a component of Bactrim and Septra, which are commonly used to treat urinary tract infections), and nalidixic acid (trade name NegGram) another drug for urinary infections. These oxidative chemicals also include nonmedical substances, such as trinitrotoluene (TNT, an explosive), phosphine (a garlicky-smelling insecticide), toluidine blue (a biological dye) and constituents of fava beans (a staple of Middle Eastern and Mediterranean cuisine).

If these oxidative substances are so dangerous, why are we all not dead from being exposed to them at one time or another?

The answer lies in yet another protective chemical system that evolution has devised for the red cell. The trick for avoiding damage by oxidative substances is getting rid of hydrogen peroxide. This is done with an enzyme called peroxidase, which converts hydrogen peroxide to harmless water. In doing so, peroxidase has to donate an electron to hydrogen peroxide. Since an enzyme is a catalyst and by definition cannot be permanently altered as a result of the reaction it presides over, it cannot donate one of its own electrons. It has to obtain an electron from another molecule called glutathione. This leaves glutathione minus one electron, which it needs to recoup if it is to participate in any further detoxifications of hydrogen peroxide. It gets this electron by stripping one from yet another molecule called NADPH. Obviously, this robbing-Peter-to-pay-Paul imbroglio has to end somewhere, and the buck stops with NADPH, a molecule that can be generated only by the breakdown of sugar by a metabolic pathway in the red cell. This metabolic pathway is presided over by an enzyme called *glucose-6-phosphate dehydrogenase*, or G6PD (fig. 6.1).

G6PD is a protein, as are all enzymes, and as such it is the product of a gene. If an individual inherits a mutated, faulty version of this gene, there is diminished ability to generate NADPH, leading to inability to generate active glutathione, causing failure of peroxidase to detoxify hydrogen peroxide, causing accumulation of free radicals, causing destruction of the red cells, which is manifested as hemolytic anemia. So, the bottom line is that if you have no G6PD, or an insufficient amount, you suffer from a hemolytic anemia that is made worse by exposure to oxidative substances. Thus G6PD deficiency can be defined as *the typically episodic hemolytic anemia resulting from an inherited deficiency in G6PD.*

Unlike all the other genes discussed here, the gene for G6PD is located on the X chromosome. Of course, males have only one X chromosome, while females have two. Furthermore, a female with at least one normal G6PD gene can make sufficient amounts of G6PD to avoid symptomatic G6PD deficiency, even

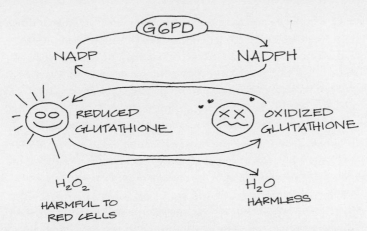

FIG. 6.I. The ability of the red cell to detoxify hydrogen peroxide (H_2O_2) is ultimately dependent on the enzyme G6PD.

if her other gene produces absolutely no G6PD. (An exception is that sometimes a woman with one normal and one mutated gene can have a mild case of G6PD deficiency, which occurs because, in early embryonic life, the normal genes in some of her cells were inactivated. This is an example of what geneticists call the Lyon hypothesis.) The unfortunate male, however, has only one X chromosome, so if he inherits a bad G6PD gene from his mother, there is no normal gene to balance it (if he had also inherited a normal G6PD gene from his father, he would, of course, not be a "he," but a "she"). G6PD deficiency can occur in females, but it is much less common, because they must have the bad luck of inheriting one bad gene from each parent.

As with thalassemia, different genes for G6PD deficiency have varying degrees of severity. Individuals with the most severe variants, which are found most commonly in Mediterranean peoples, may have a constant severe hemolytic anemia from birth. This can be mistaken clinically for alloimmune hemolytic disease of the newborn (see chapter 5). More commonly the mutated gene results in a milder deficiency manifested as episodes of hemolysis that punctuate an otherwise normal existence. These episodes are initiated by stressful stimuli, which include not only the drugs and other chemicals already mentioned, but acute infections and severe diabetic attacks (diabetic ketoacidosis). These milder levels of G6PD deficiency are especially common in African Americans, among whom 12 percent of males carry the gene. This is important for physicians to know, as it provides a ready explanation for an otherwise puzzling hemolytic episode in a previously healthy black person. (Even though the condition is much more common in males, females are likelier to experience hemolysis requiring medical attention. This is because the substances that most frequently cause hemolysis are drugs used to treat urinary tract infections, and women are much more susceptible to these infections than men.)

The treatment of G6PD deficiency hinges upon recognition that the condition exists so that the person can simply avoid oxidative substances. Newborns with severe forms of the disease may need exchange transfusions to rid the blood of toxic bilirubin, but, unlike the situation with thalassemia major, the hemolytic anemia is usually not severe enough to necessitate lifelong transfusions.

HEREDITARY SPHEROCYTOSIS

The abnormalities covered so far in this chapter (except for G6PD deficiency) have been the result of mutated genes that code for the globin protein subunits of hemoglobin. Although this book has concentrated on the role of red cells in the production and maintenance of hemoglobin, the DNA of the developing red cells is responsible for cellular proteins other than hemoglobin and the enzymes that keep it happy. For instance, the normal shape of the RBC, referred to as a biconcave disk (a round-edged disk with dented-in top and bottom), is not the natural shape of a bag of fluid. If you take an infinitely flexible, elastic closed bag and fill it with any fluid, it will naturally form a perfect sphere. (We can easily demonstrate this concept in the real world by blowing soap bubbles.) Red cells are also bags of fluid, so any shape they maintain other than a sphere is due to some degree of rigidity of the membranes that enclose them. (Rigidity is a relative term here; obviously, red cells are not as rigid as wood or metal.)

The biconcave shape of the RBC is maintained by a lattice of proteins lying immediately beneath the cell membrane. This network of girder-like molecules is called the cytoskeleton; it vaguely resembles the cage structure of one of R. Buckminster Fuller's geodesic domes. Each girder consists of a protein molecule called spectrin. Spectrin is anchored to the red cell membrane by another protein, ankyrin, and a host of other proteins are involved as well. If the gene coding for spectrin, or ankyrin, or other associated cytoskeletal proteins is defective by way of a mutation, spectrin will not be found in normal amounts in the structure. As with the removal of successive girders from a geodesic dome, leaving out just a few spectrin molecules will have little observable effect on the structure of the cell. As more girders are removed, the structure becomes successively weaker and eventually gives way to whatever physical forces act on it. With a geodesic sphere, that force is gravity, and the dome collapses. In the case of the RBC, that force is the surface tension of the cell membrane. Surface tension acts to draw up the spectrin-deficient, weak-walled red cell into a sphere called, appropriately enough, a spherocyte.

As red cells go, spherocytes are not all that bad. Hemoglobin is just as happy living in a spherical house as a biconcave one, and spherocytes have no trouble negotiating the cramped quarters of the microcirculation. The spleen, however, is not amused. Bringing McCarthyism to the cellular level, this most arbitrary organ will have nothing of a nonconformist spherical red cell and will summarily execute the offender once the latter is trapped in the splenic sinusoids. This results in decreased red cell survival, and, if the marrow cannot produce enough red cells to compensate for the slaughter, the result is hemolytic anemia. This leads us to the definition of hereditary spherocytosis (HS):

*the congenital hemolytic anemia resulting from splenic removal
of red cells with an abnormal spherical shape due to an inherited
defect in cytoskeleton structure.*

The inherited hemolytic anemias discussed so far
(hemoglobinopathies and thalassemias) are far more common
in dark-skinned races than in fair-skinned peoples of northern
European heritage. Hereditary spherocytosis is the just the
opposite. In fact, HS is the most common cause of inherited
hemolytic anemia among Americans of northern European
descent. The actual gene frequency in this population is about
I percent, but the majority of these cases have such a mild
abnormality that there are no problems and the condition is
never discovered. HS is different from hemoglobinopathies and
thalassemias is another fundamental way. The latter are *recessive*;
that is, the adverse effect of the abnormal gene inherited from
one parent is ameliorated by the effect of the normal gene
inherited from the other. In sickle cell trait, for instance, while
the bad gene makes hemoglobin S, the good gene makes enough
hemoglobin A to keep the red cells from sickling or hemolyzing.
In contrast, HS is *dominant*, meaning that the bad gene inherited
from one parent does enough harm to interfere with the normal
function of the good gene. Accordingly, inheriting just one HS
gene is enough to cause a hemolytic anemia. Anyone unfortunate
enough to inherit a double dose of the HS gene may be visited
with a severe hemolytic anemia. Fortunately, this is rare.

There are many genetic diseases in the field of hematology
and in every other subspecialty of medicine, and trying to
remember which are recessive and which are dominant can
drive medical students crazy. I had this problem for years, until
I ran into a valuable rule of thumb. If the bad gene codes
for a *functional* protein molecule (like a globin subunit or an
enzyme), it is usually a recessive trait. If the bad gene codes for a
structural protein molecule (like ankyrin or spectrin), it is usually
dominant. Like every rule, this one has its exceptions, but it is
easier to memorize those than to try to remember every single
item on two very long lists.

As with beta-thalassemia, there are numerous different mutations, resulting in a wide spectrum of clinical severity. Fortunately, the vast majority of HS cases are fairly mild. While these people do have hemolytic anemia for life, few require transfusion after the neonatal period. The biggest problem they have is gallstones, because lifelong hemolysis means lifelong overproduction of bilirubin. Bilirubin, which is a solid dissolved in a liquid (bile), can crystallize out of solution if present in higher than normal concentrations. This occurs in the gallbladder, which is nothing but a bile-filled pouch hanging from the bile duct system. The crystals of bilirubin are microscopic at first, but they eventually build up into stones measuring millimeters to centimeters in diameter. The stones can cause the typical abdominal pain of a "gallbladder attack," which is classically described as beginning in the right upper portion of the abdomen and radiating to the back or shoulder. Stones can also get squeezed out of the gallbladder, where they can lodge in the common bile duct, blocking the secretion of bile and causing a severe degree of jaundice. Blockage also interferes with excretion of another component of bile, bile salts, which are the detergent-like ingredients that allow fat to be digested in the small bowel. This results not only in malabsorption of fats in the diet but also in the buildup of bile acids in the blood and tissues. Bile acids are especially irritating to the skin and produce a maddening state of constant itching all over the body. The most feared complication of bile duct obstruction is acute bacterial infection of the bile duct, or *ascending cholangitis*, which can be life threatening.

The diagnosis of hereditary spherocytosis begins with the diagnosis of hemolytic anemia, as discussed in chapter 5. Examination of the blood smear may show the characteristic spherocytes, but in some cases this finding is so subtle that it can be missed. Fortunately there is another lab test for detecting spherocytes, the osmotic fragility test. To understand how it works, we have to take yet another detour into basic cell biology.

With a few rather important exceptions (the skin cells, for instance), cell membranes do not present any kind of impediment to the passage of water. Water follows the law of mass action (mentioned in Chapter I in the discussion of oxygen transport by hemoglobin). This means that water will move across a cell membrane from the side with the greater concentration of water to the side with the lesser concentration of water. Pure water has a greater concentration than water containing dissolved solids, so water normally moves from compartments with a low concentration of dissolved solids to those with high concentrations of the same. Red cells normally float in plasma, which contains salt at a concentration of 0.9 percent (roughly ⅓ that of open seawater). To safely taste this for yourself, you can simulate the saltiness of plasma by mixing up some normal saline solution in the kitchen; just dissolve ¼ teaspoon table salt in 10 ounces of tap water.

If you were to take normal red cells, spin them down in a centrifuge, pour off the plasma, and resuspend them in some of your homemade normal saline, they would float around and live for a few hours (until they ran out of oxygen and nutrients), all the while maintaining their normal biconcave shape. If, however, you were to resuspend them in a solution that had only half the concentration of salt that was in your normal saline solution, then water would flow across the cell membrane into the cell, which has a higher concentration of salt than does the surrounding solution. This causes the cell to swell up and the biconcave disk shape to be lost, with the red cell eventually assuming a spherical shape. As you reduce the salt concentration of the external solution further, the cell becomes so turgid that the cell membrane gives way, and the RBC pops, or lyses. Since the normal red cell has more membrane surface area than volume, it can withstand this osmotic stress better than a spherocyte can, which, because of its spherical shape, already has as much volume as its cell membrane can enclose. When a spherocyte is subjected to decreasing concentrations of salt, it pops sooner. While this has no bearing on the lysis of red cells in the body, the behavior of cells in artificial salt solutions can be used to detect whether a red cell has a more spherical shape than a normal cell. This is the osmotic fragility test, and it is the main lab test for spherocytosis.

Those of religious turn will be delighted to discover that the cure for hereditary spherocytosis is prescribed in the New Testament: "And if thine eye offend thee, pluck it out, and cast it from thee" (Matthew 18: 9). In this case, the offender is the spleen, and it is the surgeon who plucks and casts it out. Of course, a splenectomy is major surgery, but young healthy patients generally tolerate the procedure well. The patient does lose some of the shield against infection provided by the spleen. Fortunately, there is a vaccine against the *pneumococcus* bacterium, which at one time was a frequent cause of life-threatening infections in people without spleens. This vaccine *must be given* to anyone who is about to have the operation. Splenectomy does not cause any change in the spherocyte itself; it simply keeps a funny-looking but perfectly useful cell from meeting an untimely end at the hands of an intolerant inquisitor. Hereditary spherocytosis remains the only primary hematological disease that is uniformly curable by surgery.

IN SUMMARY

Hemoglobinopathies are inherited conditions in which a mutated gene produces globin chains with abnormal structure. The most important hemoglobinopathy is sickle cell disease, which features not only hemolytic anemia, but also episodes of blockage of blood circulation by the sickled cells, causing pain and tissue destruction. Hemoglobin C disease, found almost exclusively in blacks, is a hemolytic anemia without sickling phenomena. Hemoglobin E disease is found in Southeast Asians and results in a microcytic anemia, because the abnormal gene does not allow globin to be synthesized at a normal rate.

Thalassemias are inherited conditions characterized by an imbalance of synthesis of alpha and beta hemoglobin chain. There is wide variation in clinical severity of the various thalassemias. The most common mutation is the alpha-thalassemia variant seen in blacks, which is almost always clinically insignificant and undetected. The most severe form is the alpha-thalassemia variant seen in Asians, which when fully expressed is invariably fatal before or soon after birth. Among the beta-thalassemias, thal major is a debilitating life-shortening disease requiring lifelong transfusions and chelation therapy. Thal minor, on the other hand, causes only mild anemia and rarely requires treatment. Thalassemia minor and hemoglobin E disease are often misdiagnosed as iron deficiency anemia.

G6PD deficiency is caused by a mutated gene on the X chromosome. It leaves the red cell with inadequate capabilities for detoxifying a variety of oxidant substances, including drugs commonly used for urinary tract infections. Exposure to such a substance causes an episode of hemolysis. A mild variant of this condition is common in black populations, including African Americans. A severe variant is seen in whites of Mediterranean descent.

Hereditary spherocytosis is a genetically dominant abnormality seen in whites of northern European ancestry. It is characterized by a deficiency in the RBC cytoskeleton, resulting in red cells that have a spherical shape. These spherocytes are not tolerated by the spleen, which destroys them, causing hemolytic anemia. Surgical removal of the spleen is curative.

7. Miscellaneous Anemias

This chapter deals with anemias that do not fit into the categories discussed so far. That these diseases are lumped together under the "miscellaneous" rubric should in no way suggest that they are unimportant. Anemia of chronic disease is one of the most common anemias encountered by the physician. Anemia of chronic renal failure is universal in those who suffer loss of kidney function. Aplastic anemia is an unpleasant and serious complication of cancer chemotherapy, and refractory anemia has silently killed many, including noted astronomer and science popularizer Carl Sagan.

APLASTIC ANEMIA

Aplastic anemia is the simplest form of anemia; it is *the condition characterized by the death of blood cell precursors (erythroblasts) in the marrow.* While the root *-plasia* (from which "plastic" comes) seems to have meanings in the medical world that are different from those of everyday language, the origin of the word belies this impression. The Greek word *plassein* means "to mold or form." Regarding plastic construction materials, the word refers to their being formed in molds. In "plastic surgery" the reference is to the shapable features of the contoured parts of the body, such as the face. In the rest of the medical vocabulary, "-plasia" is used to indicate growth and development, i.e., the "forming" of cells and tissues. In hemolytic anemias, as we saw in chapter 5, the marrow fills up with erythroblasts trying to compensate for the loss of red cells in the circulation. This response is called *erythroid hyperplasia* (*hyper-*, "too much," plus *-plasia*, "growth"). The root *-a* (or *-an* before a vowel), means "not" or "without." "Aplastic," then, means "without growth," which aptly describes what happens in the bone marrow in aplastic anemia. The blood cell precursors stop growing and dividing, and they eventually die, leaving the marrow vacant of all blood-forming tissues (the marrow does not end up totally empty; instead, fat tissue takes up the space).

In a few types of aplastic anemia, just the RBC precursors die; these are grouped under the term *pure red cell aplasia*. Most cases of aplastic anemia, though, involve loss of the *myeloblasts* (precursors of white cells) and *megakaryocytes* (which give rise to platelets), as well as erythroblasts. As would be expected, these persons suffer not only from anemia but also from low counts of platelets and white cells. Low platelet count is called thrombocytopenia and is the cause of abnormal bleeding. The low white cell count, which is especially severe in the subclass of white cells known as *neutrophils*, is called neutropenia or agranulocytosis. People with neutropenia suffer from severe infections, because they have insufficient neutrophils to attack and destroy the infecting microorganisms.

Aplastic anemia typically occurs as an acute insult; that is, something really bad happens to the marrow and wipes it out in a short period of time. Paradoxically, in aplastic anemia, the anemia itself is one of the last manifestations to develop. This is because, while the red cells live in the circulation for four months, the white cells live for just a few hours and the platelets for a couple of weeks. When the precursor cells die in the marrow, the short-lived white cells disappear in less than a day, and the platelet count falls a week or so later. Only the long-lived red cells continue to circulate for 120 days—fat, dumb, and happy—oblivious that the rustlers have burned down the family ranch back home. When the red cells are finally ready to retire, they are not replaced by the dead marrow, and anemia finally results. As might be expected, this is a *hyporegenerative*, *normocytic*, *normochromic* anemia (low reticulocyte count, normal MCV and MCHC).

There are two general categories of aplastic anemia, *idiopathic* and *secondary*. Idiopathic aplastic anemias have no identifiable cause. About all we can say now is that the injury that causes the damage is on the gene, not unlike that which causes leukemia. Some cases of aplastic anemia are eventually followed by the development of leukemia in the same person. While leukemia, which is the uncontrolled proliferation of blood cell precursors in the marrow, may seem like the antithesis of aplasia, both diseases kill by destroying normal, functional blood cells.

Idiopathic aplastic anemia may occur at any age, but the elderly are most often affected. It is interesting that in Japan and other parts of East Asia, aplastic anemia is more common than in the U.S. and Europe. Conversely, leukemia is more common here than in Asia. The reason for this epidemiologic split is not known, but apparently environmental, not hereditary, factors are at work.

Secondary aplastic anemias are those for which some identifiable cause is observed. The most common example is the marrow injury that occurs as a result of cancer chemotherapy. Over the past three decades, oncologists, the doctors who treat cancer, have made such developments in the art and science of chemotherapy that severe, irreversible aplastic anemia is rare. Much more frightening are the cases that appear after exposures to occupational hazards and normally harmless drugs.

The classic occupational cause of aplastic anemia, fortunately not seen anymore, was radium. Between 1908 and the late 1920s, the numerals on the faces of some timepieces were painted with a mixture of radium sulfate and zinc sulfide. The radium, with its 1620-year half-life, provided permanent luminescence through its excitement of the fluorescent zinc sulfide by high-energy radiation. The unfortunate dial painters, mostly young women, ingested the radium dust by licking their paintbrushes to fashion a sharp point for fine lettering. Radium, which the body thinks is calcium (the two elements are chemically similar), is naively deposited in the bone by the cells charged with maintaining and repairing the skeleton. The marrow eventually becomes encased in radioactive bone. The radiation kills the blood-forming cells, and aplastic anemia is the result. Ingested radium is so dangerous that it and its radioactive cousin, plutonium, are widely considered to be the deadliest poisons known. The lethal dose is on the order of ten millionths of a gram.

The most important occupational cause of aplastic anemia is benzene. This is a hydrocarbon (an organic compound consisting of only carbon and hydrogen atoms) widely used in the chemical industry. Benzene was once a major component of a wide variety of solvents, but in many applications it has been replaced by less toxic substances. Although its harmful effect on the marrow was first noticed as early as 1897, benzene continues to enjoy a prominent place in industry and is considered an irreplaceable chemical in many applications. Because of modern workplace safety standards, the level of exposure is low enough to avoid toxicity. Fortunately, benzene is a highly odoriferous chemical, and the levels at which it can be perceived by the human nose are far lower than those that would harm the marrow. If you don't smell any benzene, then you don't have to worry about it. Benzene is the only hydrocarbon solidly linked with aplastic anemia; the scores of other such chemicals, including most modern paint thinners, kerosene, and petroleum ether, have shown no adverse effects on blood-forming cells. Modern motor fuels used in America contain 1 to 2 percent benzene, so gasoline and similar chemicals should be handled with respect, but not fear.

Therapeutic drugs that normally do not harm the marrow can rarely cause a total wipeout of blood cell precursors. This type of unpredictable damage, which is not related to the amount of the drug given, is called an idiosyncratic side effect, in contrast to the marrow injury caused by radiation and anticancer drugs, which is an example of a dose-dependent side effect. Although over 40 drugs have been implicated as culprits, the classic idiosyncratic drug-related aplastic anemia is caused by the antibiotic chloramphenicol. Although rare (1 case of aplasia per 20,000 to 30,000 uses of the drug), this side effect is of sufficient gravity to warrant care in the use of chloramphenicol. While indispensable for treating certain infections (especially meningitis in young children), chloramphenicol is now used for only a very few diseases.

Viral infections are notorious for causing bouts of marrow aplasia. Most of these episodes are limited to a few days, and the marrow recovers fully. Since red cells have a long life span in the blood, a factory shutdown for a small fraction of that time has no demonstrable effect on the red cell counts. It is a different story for those with chronic hemolytic anemias, such as hereditary spherocytosis and sickle cell disease. Their red cells are so short-lived that brisk, constant replacement is necessary to maintain reasonable RBC counts. A marrow shutdown for a few days can result in a precipitous fall in the number of circulating red cells. In people with sickle cell, this is called *aplastic crisis*, a complication to add to the other unpleasant acute episodes that beset those with the disease.

Some cases of aplastic anemia resolve on their own. For those that do not, the only hope for a permanent cure at this time is a bone marrow transplant. This is a heroic medical procedure of epic proportions, but it has resulted in apparent cures in as many as 70 percent of the patients on whom it has been tried. The key to a successful marrow transplant is obtaining a donor whose tissues most perfectly match those of the intended recipient. In most cases, such good matches can only be found in the person's siblings. For those who have no sibling matches, other blood relatives can be tested for compatibility. Efforts have been directed at developing large computer databases of donor volunteers for transplantation to nonrelatives. Since the probability of a perfect match between two unrelated individuals is 1 in 40,000, such databases have to be huge. Moreover, it is difficult to get people to agree to donate marrow to someone other than a loved one, because the procedure involves much more time, pain, risk, and inconvenience than are called for in giving a pint of blood at the local blood center.

The marrow transplant begins by treating the aplastic anemia patient with large doses of cancer chemotherapy drugs and radiation in an effort to kill off any immune system cells that may try to attack the donated marrow, mistaking it for a foreign invader. As an added benefit, the drugs and radiation treatments destroy the few remaining blood-forming cells in the patient's marrow. Since these genetically damaged cells may eventually give rise to leukemia, it is best to dispense with them permanently. The next step is to harvest from the volunteer donor about one liter of marrow, which has to be sucked out through wide-bore needles inserted into the pelvic bones. Because only a few milliliters of marrow can be removed from each site, over a hundred separate sticks have to be performed. Even so saintly a soul as a marrow donor could not withstand this torture, so he or she has to be put under general anesthesia in an operating room. The marrow, which is like a thin, bloody soup with little chunks of tissue floating around in it, is passed through a series of fine metal screens, a process which homogenizes it and yields a uniform suspension of blood-forming cells. The marrow need not be sent directly into the recipient's bone but is simply injected intravenously. The blood-forming cells will find their way to the marrow and take up residence on their own. If all goes well, the recipient's entire immune system and blood-forming tissue will, within a few months, be composed entirely of healthy cells derived from the donor tissues.

ANEMIA OF CHRONIC RENAL FAILURE

In our discussion of hemolytic anemias, we noted that the marrow responds to accelerated RBC destruction by turning out red cells at a faster rate. What we did not mention was how the marrow "knows" to turn up cell production. The chemical message sent as a wake-up call to the marrow originates from, of all places, the kidneys! Better known for their role as eliminators of chemical wastes, these two bean-shaped organs have a less glamorous role as secretors of the hormone erythropoietin. The kidneys are capable of detecting anemia and responding to a drop in hemoglobin with an increase in the release of erythropoietin into the blood. The erythropoietin stimulates red cell precursors in the marrow to put up or shut up.

Chronic renal failure (CRF) describes a progressive destruction of kidney tissues accompanied by loss of kidney function. CRF can be caused by a variety of diseases, including diabetes, hypertension, atherosclerosis, bacterial infections, and lupus, but many cases are of unknown cause. As the excretory function of kidneys is lost, natural toxins build up and cause numerous biochemical abnormalities throughout the body, a condition called uremia. Uremia can be successfully managed for long periods of time by dialysis, the use of artificial kidneys to periodically cleanse the blood. From the hematologic standpoint, the problem with dialysis is that it can only eliminate what the kidney ordinarily disposes of; it cannot *replace* what that organ normally produces. As more and more of the patient's kidney is destroyed, the production of erythropoietin drops until there is no stimulation of the marrow to compensate for anemia. The patient with fully developed renal failure, then, ends up with a chronic *hyporegenerative, normocytic, normochromic anemia.* The hemoglobin usually ranges between 5 and 7 grams per deciliter in CRF patients.

In the past, those who suffered from chronic renal failure had to manage with their low hemoglobins and accept the occasional transfusion when needed. Clearly, erythropoietin would provide effective treatment, but for decades after this hormone was identified, it could not be manufactured for pharmaceutical use. A great breakthrough came in 1985, when the human gene that codes for erythropoietin was inserted into hamster ovary cells. These nonhuman cells, grown in laboratory dishes, produced erythropoietin that was just as "human" as that produced by our own healthy kidneys. This recombinant erythropoietin, marketed under the trade name Epogen, became available commercially in 1989. It is now approved by the U.S. Food and Drug Administration for treatment of the anemia of chronic renal failure. Since this drug is a protein-like molecule, it cannot be taken by mouth without being digested and destroyed in the digestive tract but must be given by either intravenous or subcutaneous injection. The latter method, which involves a thin needle being inserted just under the skin, can be performed by patients themselves (as diabetics give themselves insulin). Some find the subcutaneous injections painful and prefer to receive the drug through an IV at the dialysis center. The favorable effect of erythropoietin injections on the quality of life for a CRF patient is remarkable. The availability of this drug has cut the need for blood transfusions by a factor of ten.

The CRF patient's ultimate leap to freedom comes in the form of a kidney transplant. Those who are fortunate enough to receive this priceless gift are also relieved of their anemia, as the properly functioning transplanted kidney is perfectly capable of synthesizing and secreting erythropoietin.

REFRACTORY ANEMIA

"Refractory," deriving from a Latin word meaning "stubborn," is an appropriate descriptive term for this condition. To some extent, refractory anemia (RA) resembles megaloblastic anemia, in that it is characteristically a *hyporegenerative, macrocytic, normochromic anemia* (low reticulocyte count, high MCV, normal MCHC). There are other similarities as well, including the frequent concurrence of low counts of circulating white blood cells and platelets. When these counts are low and anemia is present, the term applied is *pancytopenia (pan + cyto + penia = all + cells + deficient)*. The similarity ends there, since RA cannot be corrected by administration of B$_{12}$ or folate. Because this condition stubbornly fails to respond to any of the *hematinic* ("blood-building") vitamins or iron, the term "refractory" was adopted.

Refractory anemia is now known to be caused by damage to the DNA of developing blood cells in the bone marrow. The marrow fills up with blood cell precursors, but they cannot get out into the bloodstream. This is another example of ineffective erythropoiesis, as seen in beta-thalassemia major and megaloblastic anemias, except that the disease mechanisms behind these conditions are different. The genetic material in the blood-producing cells of RA patients is so unstable that 15 percent of these individuals eventually develop acute leukemia, an aggressive cancer of the blood-forming cells with a very poor prognosis. For this reason, RA is grouped with several other similar hematological conditions under the rubric *preleukemic syndromes* or *myelodysplastic syndromes.*

Typically, refractory anemia develops in older people, although no age group is immune. The diagnosis is suspected when an older person shows pancytopenia and normal serum B_{12} and folate levels. Some physicians may try a course of B_{12} and folate therapy to confirm that the anemia is indeed refractory. At this point, most physicians will refer the person for a bone marrow biopsy (see appendix D). This is done to rule out other causes of hyporegenerative pancytopenia, including aplastic anemia (discussed above), various types of cancer, and other, more aggressive preleukemic syndromes. The biopsy is also an opportunity to obtain a specimen for analysis of the chromosomes in the abnormal cells. Some chromosomal abnormalities have prognostic significance.

The anemia of RA can be treated by blood transfusion. Things get worse for the patient when the platelet and white cell counts drop to dangerous levels, causing bleeding and severe infections, respectively. Although platelets can be transfused, their shorter life span means that the procedure must be done more frequently than with red cell transfusions. Eventually, the person develops antibodies to the donor platelets, and subsequent transfusions are ineffective. White cell transfusions are theoretically available, but they are impractical for long-term use. The only hope for a cure is a marrow transplant, but, because of the advanced age of most RA patients, this measure is feasible in less than 10 percent of the cases. The average survival time after diagnosis of RA is about 2½ years. The most common immediate cause of death is infection.

ANEMIA OF CHRONIC DISEASE

Even though anemia of chronic disease is the second most common anemia (after iron deficiency), discussion of it has been saved for last. This is because there is no diagnostic test for anemia of chronic disease, the result being a *diagnosis of exclusion*, meaning that the diagnosis is made only after it has been established that all of the other forms of anemia have been eliminated as possibilities. Consideration of this anemia is best put at the end also because of the mystery surrounding it, as we shall see.

Briefly defined, anemia of chronic disease (ACD) is *that anemia which accompanies general systemic illnesses, especially those characterized by inflammation.* The underlying disease can be any from a long list of chronic ailments, including infections, collagen-vascular diseases (such as lupus and rheumatoid arthritis), and cancer (even though a cancerous tumor is not an inflammatory process, the body's immune system may react to the tumor with some manifestations of the inflammatory response). Under our cytometric classification, ACD is a *hyporegenerative normocytic/microcytic, normochromic/hypochromic* anemia. This means that the reticulocyte count is low, the MCV is normal or low, and the MCHC is normal or low. Before going into more detail, let us consider the inflammatory response; for this we have to break away from our exclusive interest in the red cell and visit the even more complex world of the white cell.

White cells, or leukocytes, are the individual instruments in the great symphony that is the immune response. There are three major types of leukocytes involved in the inflammatory response, all of which not only circulate in the blood, but also reside and work in the solid tissues throughout the body. These major categories of white cells are neutrophils, monocytes, and lymphocytes.

Neutrophils, the most numerous of the circulating white cells, are considered the shock troops of the inflammatory response. When a microbial invader enters a normally sterile area of the body, millions of neutrophils accumulate at the site and attempt to destroy the invader by engulfing it and exposing it to an armamentarium of highly toxic substances. In the process of doing this, the neutrophils also fall victim to their own weapons. The innumerable dead neutrophils pile up and break down, to the point where their mass grave becomes visible to the naked eye as a creamy yellow material, called pus. One of the deadly chemicals produced by these turned-on neutrophils before they die is an iron-containing substance called lactoferrin. When the inflammatory response is activated, neutrophils respond by markedly increasing their synthesis of lactoferrin and secreting it into the plasma (more on this later).

Monocytes, the least numerous of the three main leukocyte types, circulate around in the blood until they are needed at the battlefield to combat an unfriendly microbe. When they leave the circulation and enter the tissues, they transform into macrophages. (Remember from chapter 5 that macrophages are also a part of the reticuloendothelial system, charged with getting rid of aged red cells and readily scarfing up red cells coated with antibodies.) Macrophages are equally enthusiastic about engulfing and destroying infectious agents, especially those that are coated with antibodies. Another function of macrophages is to take some of these engulfed organisms and "present" them to the cells that actually make the antibodies. You can think of the macrophage as the big goon who picks up the trouble-making punk by the collar, drags him before the local kingpin, Mr. Lymphocyte (see below), and then beats up his hapless victim at the behest of the boss.

Another function of macrophages in the marrow is to store iron and transfer it to developing red cell precursors for hemoglobin production. For the marrow macrophages to get their iron in the first place, they have to receive it from transferrin, the major iron transport protein in the blood. In conditions where the immune response is turned on, much of the lactoferrin produced by the neutrophils ends up going into the macrophages. Presumably this lactoferrin will be put to good use by the macrophages out on the battlefield, because lactoferrin is quite capable of killing bacteria. Back home in the marrow, however, the lactoferrin competes with transferrin for receptor sites on the macrophages. The iron in lactoferrin is not available for transfer to developing red cells, so these go hungry, while more and more iron is piling up unused in the macrophages. The result is that, in ACD, the amount of storage iron is increased, but the transfer of that iron to erythroblasts is blocked. This explains why some cases of ACD resemble iron deficiency to the extent that the red cells are small and pale. In true iron deficiency anemia, of course, storage iron is absent. Because of the marked difference between iron deficiency and ACD in respect to the disposition of iron, evaluation of the amount of storage iron in a marrow biopsy can be a very valuable test in distinguishing between the two conditions.

Lymphocytes are the second most numerous of the three major types of white cells. They not only circulate in the blood but also reside in large numbers in so-called "lymphoid tissues" throughout the body. The classic example of lymphoid tissue is the lymph nodes, which are solid packages of lymphocytes. Other prominent areas of lymphoid tissue are found in the upper throat and digestive tract.

If the neutrophils and monocytes are the brawny enforcers in the war on microbes, then the lymphocytes are the brains. These little cells cannot engulf bacteria and other germs directly, but they can perform two other functions that are just as deadly. First, one class of lymphocytes, called B cells, can produce antibodies specific to the molecules sticking out on the surface of the invader. When functioning properly, these antibodies stick only onto those specific molecules that signify an enemy. Macrophages and neutrophils respond to the antibody tag by eating whatever the tag is attached to and leaving untagged cells alone. This is why the immune response can kill outsiders while leaving our own tissues untouched. The second deadly weapon at the lymphocyte's command is the lymphokines, a motley assemblage of substances secreted by lymphocytes involved in the inflammatory/immune response. Lymphokines act as intermediaries among lymphocytes, variously hiking up and toning down inflammatory activity so as to meet infectious threats with measured response and minimal collateral damage. Several of these lymphokines have the property of being able to inhibit cell growth. The influence of these cells on erythroblasts is to make them less responsive to erythropoietin stimulation. The effects of this growth-inhibiting property of lymphokines are not limited to RBC precursors; other cells are similarly affected. For instance, during periods of acute or chronic inflammation, nails and hair also grow more slowly. Finally, some lymphokines inhibit the excretion of erythropoietin by the kidney, further enhancing the slowdown of red cell production.

As a result of the combined effect of these manifestations of the inflammatory response, anemia of chronic disease is characterized by:

(1) Accumulation of iron in macrophages, causing lack of iron for hemoglobin synthesis.

(2) Decreased responsiveness of red cells to erythropoietin stimulation.

(3) Decreased production of erythropoietin by the kidney.

From the above, it is easy to see how a hyporegenerative anemia can develop, and how such an anemia may impersonate iron deficiency by showing microcytosis and hypochromia. Another phenomenon reflecting the hoarding of iron by macrophages is that the serum iron level is typically low, as in iron deficiency. Unlike iron deficiency, which is characterized by a compensatory increase in transferrin in the serum, ACD is accompanied by a *decrease* in transferrin (or, as is measured in many labs, total iron binding capacity, TIBC). The serum ferritin, which is an indirect reflection of body iron stores, is elevated as expected (cf. iron deficiency, in which ferritin is low).

The diagnosis of anemia of chronic disease is usually straightforward, but does require clinical judgement and a few strategically selected lab tests. Typically the patient has a history of some chronic disease. The hemoglobin is low, but usually above 10 grams per deciliter. The reticulocyte count is low. Serum iron and transferrin/TIBC are low, but ferritin is high. Rarely it may be necessary to perform a bone marrow biopsy to assess iron stores, but this is necessary only in complex or confusing cases (for instance, just because a patient has a chronic disease does not mean iron deficiency anemia could not also occur as the result of a bleeding ulcer or other significant abnormality).

A summary of typical lab test results in ACD is given in the following table. This should be compared with the similar table in chapter 3.

Test	Expected Result
hemoglobin	low
MCV	normal or low
MCHC	normal or low
serum iron	low
serum transferrin (or TIBC)	low
per cent iron saturation	normal
serum ferritin	high

Anemia of chronic disease is usually so mild that it does not require treatment. Cases severe enough to cause symptoms may respond to injections of recombinant erythropoietin. Doctors mainly need to know what *not* to do in treatment of ACD: blood transfusions should almost never be used, and oral or injectable iron should not be given.

Appendices

APPENDIX A:
A Mercifully Brief Note on the Metric System

Americans remain the only industrialized people on earth who are intimidated by the metric system. I am not going to scare the reader off with a complex, fine-print conversion table, but, since the study of anemia is meaningless without some appreciation for the measurement of the physical properties of blood, I offer the following information.

The *gram* is the metric unit of *mass*, which for our purposes is the same as weight. One dry ounce is about 28 grams. Prefixes are used to denote minute fractions of a gram; thus, one thousandth of a gram is a *milligram*, one millionth of a gram is a *microgram*, one billionth is a *nanogram*, and one trillionth is a *picogram*. We could list how many picograms are in an ounce, but the number of zeros would be deadening to the senses, and such a figure is a total abstraction with no meaning in the sensorial world. It is best just to accept these impossibly tiny quantities as numbers and not to worry about how small a fraction of a bushel they are.

The *liter* is the metric unit of *volume* and is a bit more than a U.S. quart. One thousandth of a liter is a *milliliter*, which for our purposes is exactly the same as a cubic centimeter (referred to in every medical TV show that ever aired as a "cc"). Since no one can say "milliliter" without getting tongue-tied, we refer to "mL" by pronouncing the letters ("em-ell"), or just say "mill" for short. There are about 30 mL in a fluid ounce, 15 mL in a tablespoonful, and 5 mL in a teaspoonful. We can also use the same prefixes we used for grams to refer to tiny fractions of a liter; hence, a *microliter* is a millionth of a liter, a *nanoliter* is a billionth, a *picoliter* is a trillionth, and a *femtoliter* is a quadrillionth. For some reason, a microliter is referred to as a "lambda." As with minuscule fractions of grams, such tiny portions of a liter are completely outside human experience and are best considered as pure abstractions.

In one of the convenient match-ups of the metric system, a milliliter of water weighs almost exactly 1 gram. Since most other body fluids, including blood, are over 90 percent water, this equivalence between gram and milliliter holds roughly true for them, too.

APPENDIX B:
A Whirlwind Review of Basic Cell Biology

To use this book, it is necessary to have an *understanding* of basic biology at the high school level. This means that if you just *took* high school biology, but didn't *pay attention* to it, you may have trouble. To spare you the humiliation of admitting to yourself that you had things other than school on your mind at age 16, I have included a brief review of basic cell biology.

All life on earth is based on cells. Every organism consists of 1 or more cells, each of which has some or all of the biochemical capabilities for sustaining life. Animal cells are enclosed by a thin, flexible *cell membrane* composed of protein and lipid (fat). Water passes freely through the membranes of most cells, but other substances may be held back by various chemical barriers. The portion of the cell lying within the membrane consists of the *nucleus* and the *cytoplasm*. The nucleus, which is enclosed in its own membrane, contains almost all the genetic material in the cell. This material is deoxyribonucleic acid (DNA) and consists of long chains of repeating sequences of 4 relatively small molecules called *nucleotides*. The long chains line up in pairs and twist around each other to make the famous double helix. The nucleotides are arranged in such a way as to indicate specific codes for the assembly of proteins. Each DNA sequence that codes for a given protein is called a *gene*. The DNA does not consist of 1 long chain. Instead, the genetic material of each cell is distributed among 46 separate lengths of DNA, called *chromosomes*. At the time of cell reproduction, by which 1 cell splits in 2, the chromosomes tightly wind up into short, stout rods that easily separate from each other as the cell divides.

When division is finished, and the cell is to go about its business, the chromosomes unwind to form long, tangled, vermicelli-like strands that are homogeneously distributed throughout the nucleus. Genes work by acting as templates for the assembly of proteins. This is done through an intermediary molecule, called ribonucleic acid (RNA). RNA is also composed of a repeating coded sequence of nucleotides. One form of RNA, *messenger RNA*, assembles itself along the DNA gene in the nucleus, a process called *transcription*. The messenger RNA leaves the nucleus and travels to the cytoplasm, where it is met by three-nucleotide units of *transfer RNA*. Each transfer RNA unit has attached to itself a specific amino acid. The transfer RNA units link up along the chain of messenger RNA, dragging their amino acids with them. This process, called *translation*, results in a chain of amino acids sequenced in a specific order as originally dictated by the DNA gene. Such a linked chain of amino acids is called a *protein*. There are two general types of proteins, *structural proteins* and *enzymes*. Structural proteins make up the physical parts of the organism, such as membranes, connective tissue fibers, and muscle fibers. Enzymes are molecules that act as catalysts in causing chemical reactions to proceed at a rate sufficient for the biochemical processes of life. Almost all chemical reactions in the body, including those that synthesize fats, proteins, carbohydrates, and DNA, are presided over by enzymes.

The cytoplasm, which envelopes the nucleus, contains a variety of structures, including *mitochondria*. These are bacteria-sized, lozenge-shaped bodies that are rich in enzymes used in the breakdown of sugar from which metabolic energy is extracted.

Mature red cells in the circulating blood contain neither mitochondria nor a nucleus. Their precursors in the marrow, however, do contain these structures. Circulating red cells cannot reproduce, and because they have no mitochondria, can generate only a meager amount of energy.

APPENDIX C:
Typical Normal Values for Common Hematologic Lab Tests

The following are normal ranges for commonly ordered laboratory tests used in the assessment of anemia. Keep in mind that these are just sample ranges from one lab, and that different labs have different reference ranges. All values given below are for adults.

Test	Normal Range	Units
RBC count, male	4.7–6.1	million/μL
RBC count, female	4.2–5.4	million/μL
Hemoglobin, male	14–18	g/dL
Hemoglobin, female	12–16	g/dL
Hematocrit, male	0.42–0.52	L/L
Hematocrit, female	0.37–0.47	L/L
MCV	80–94	fL
MCHC	32–36	g/dL
Reticulocyte count	0.5–1.5	percent

APPENDIX D: Bone Marrow Biopsy

Most anemias can be diagnosed accurately from a history, physical exam, and a few simple blood tests. But for some, such as aplastic anemia and refractory anemia, it is usually necessary to examine the blood-forming cells in the bone marrow. To sample this tissue, a bone marrow biopsy is done.

In adults, the sample is usually taken from the pelvic bone, typically from the posterior superior iliac spine (the prominence of bone on either side of the pelvis underlying the "bikini dimples" on the lower back/upper buttocks). Hematologists do bone marrow biopsies all the time, but most internists and pathologists and many family practitioners are also trained to perform the procedure.

With the patient lying face down or on the side, the skin over the biopsy site is deadened with a local anesthetic. The anesthetic needle is then inserted deeper to deaden the surface membrane covering the bone (the periosteum). Next, a larger rigid needle with a very sharp point is introduced into the marrow space. A syringe is attached to the needle and suction is applied, drawing the marrow cells into the syringe. This suction step may be uncomfortable, since it is impossible to completely deaden the inside of the bone. The contents of the syringe, which to the naked eye looks like blood with tiny chunks of fat floating around in it, is dropped onto a glass microscope slide and smeared out. After the cells are stained, they are visible to the examining pathologist or hematologist.

This part of the procedure, the *aspiration*, is usually followed by the *core biopsy*, in which a slightly larger needle is used to extract a core of bone. Even though the core biopsy procedure involves a bigger needle, it is usually less painful than the aspiration. The calcium in the bony specimen is chemically removed from the bone to make it soft, and the tissue is processed in a machine that removes all the water in the tissue, replacing it with paraffin wax. A histologic technician cuts thin ($\frac{1}{200}$ millimeter) slices of the tissue on an instrument called a microtome. The slices are picked up on glass microscope slides. The wax is dissolved, and, in a complicated series of solvents and solutions, the tissue sections are stained for examination.

Appendix E:
Mistakes Doctors Make Concerning Anemia

This is admittedly a highly editorialized section, but it is based on my observations from fifteen-plus years of general pathology practice in various academic and private venues. Others may or may not agree with these assessments, but I believe mistakes include the following:

(1) *Assuming all anemia is iron deficiency*. Most doctors do know that a man or postmenopausal woman with iron deficiency

anemia is likely to have a significant bleeding lesion of the digestive tract and to need an endoscopic evaluation. The problem is that too often the endoscopy is requested before it has been ascertained that the anemia is due to iron deficiency. An endoscopy, while relatively safe, costs thousands of dollars and is not most people's idea of a pleasant way to spend the day. Physicians should take the red cell indices and serum iron studies into account before making that diagnosis.

(2) *Assuming all microcytic, hypochromic anemia is iron deficiency.* Thalassemia minor is very common, but it does not get much press. I have seen women treated for years with iron tablets when all they have is thalassemia minor requiring no treatment (although genetic counseling is advisable). Thal minor may be difficult to diagnose, but one easy way is to bring both parents in for testing. All that needs to be done on each is a simple blood count costing less than ten dollars. If the patient has thal minor, then one of the parents should also have it, and the blood counts should reflect this (borderline low hemoglobin, disproportionately low MCV).

(3) *Getting hemoglobinopathies and thalassemias confused.* Some doctors appreciate the need to rule out thal in a patient who has a microcytic anemia. The problem is that they order a hemoglobin electrophoresis. This test is excellent for detecting some hemoglobinopathies (including hemoglobins S, C, and E), but it is usually normal in pure thalassemia. When the test comes back normal, the doctor incorrectly concludes that thalassemia has been ruled out.

(4) *Not ordering a reticulocyte count.* There are many causes of normocytic, normochromic anemia, and the quickest way to get to the diagnosis is to decide first whether a given case is a hemolytic anemia or a hyporegenerative anemia. The reticulocyte count, which is inexpensive and can be done in any laboratory, is the easiest way to accomplish this. If the patient has a hemolytic anemia, then a careful drug history, direct Coombs' test, and expert smear examination are in order. If the reticulocyte is low, a bone marrow biopsy may have to be

ordered. Therefore, the retic count is pivotal in deciding what steps are to be taken next.

(5) *Unnecessary bone marrow biopsies.* Expensive and painful, bone marrow biopsies should be reserved for anemias that cannot be explained by less invasive lines of inquiry. For instance, it is not necessary to perform a bone marrow biopsy to diagnose most cases of megaloblastic anemia, iron deficiency anemia, hemolytic anemia, and anemia of chronic disease. Too often, the primary care physician requests a bone marrow biopsy at the same time that all other tests are being ordered (the so-called "shotgun" approach). This practice would probably change if all doctors actually had to *undergo* a biopsy as part of their training.

(6) *Not paying attention to the red cell indices.* Doctors often respond to anemia by ordering serum B_{12}, folate, iron, and transferrin levels. This makes no sense, because the two diseases (iron deficiency and megaloblastic anemia) develop in different scenarios, and also because one causes little red cells and the other big ones. Clearly, someone out there is ignoring the results of the routine blood count.

(7) *Paying too much attention to pharmaceutical salespeople.* All sorts of expensive iron-replacement drugs are on the market. When I was in medical school, we were told repeatedly that almost all cases of iron deficiency respond to ferrous sulfate, the least expensive of all; twenty years later, standard textbooks still say the same thing, but those expensive iron pills continue to flow like water.

A P P E N D I X   F : Resources for Additional Information

Blood, by James H. Jandl (2nd ed., Little, Brown, and Co., 1996), is the definitive textbook on hematology and is arguably the best single-author medical textbook in print. Dr. Jandl holds the Minot professorship at Harvard Medical School, and his wit and elegance of language permeate every paragraph of this

1500-page tome. This is an upper-level medical text, requiring a fairly heavy biomedical background.

The Red Cell and Anemia has most of the information in this book in a more condensed form (about 50 pages). It is written for second-year medical students and presumes knowledge of biochemistry and physiology at the college level. It can be downloaded free from http://www.neosoft.com/~uthman/REDCELL.PDF, but requires a computer-specific Adobe Acrobat Reader application to display and print it. The free Acrobat Reader program can be downloaded from http://www.adobe.com/prodindex/acrobat/readstep.html.

Hematology: The Blossoming of a Science, by Maxwell M. Wintrobe (Lea & Febiger, 1985), is the book of choice for those who wish to learn more about the history of hematology, written by a man who is part of that history.

Lab Test Interpretation is a free encyclopedic online resource on lab tests by the author of this book. It may be accessed on the Web at http://www.neosoft.com/~uthman/lab_test.html.

The *Illustrated Guide to Diagnostic Tests* (Springhouse, 1993) does a nice job of describing all the important blood tests covered in this book, as well as most other commonly performed diagnostic tests. It is aimed at nurses, but most general readers will also benefit from its contents.

The *USDA Nutrient Database for Standard Reference* is an enormous repository of nutritional information on every imaginable foodstuff. It may be accessed online at http://www.nal.usda.gov/fnic/cgi-bin/nut_search.pl.

Understanding Sickle Cell Disease, by Miriam Bloom (University Press of Mississippi, 1995), is the first volume in this series and, like this book, is written for the general readership. A voluminous appendix lists a large number of resources for the support of sickle cell patients and their families. Dr. Bloom is a geneticist, and her excellent introduction to the genetic basis of heredity provides a serendipitous bonus.

The *Cooley's Anemia Foundation* has an excellent thalassemia page on the World Wide Web, accessible at http://pages.prodigy.com/thalassemia/. The phone number for the national office is (800) 522–7222.

The *G6PD Deficiency Home Page*, on the Web at http://rialto.com/g6pd/, has useful original information, as well as links to several informative sites concerning this condition.

The *Aplastic Anemia Foundation of America* has a World Wide Web site at http://www.teleport.com/nonprofit/aafa/index.html. Their voice phone is (800) 747–2820.

The *National Marrow Donor Program* has a Web site at http://www.marrow.org/. Their phone number is (800) MARROW-2.

Information about recombinant erythropoietin (Epogen) is available online at http://wwwext.amgen.com/cgi-bin/genobject/productEpogen. The drug's manufacturer, Amgen, can be reached by voice phone at (805) 447–1000.

The author of this book can be reached by e-mail at uthman@neosoft.com. Readers are also invited to visit his Web page at http://www.neosoft.com/~uthman/.

Glossary

Albumin The collective term used to describe a group of plasma proteins with various functions, including the transport of bilirubin from the reticuloendothelial system to the liver.

Amino acid Any one of about twenty small-to-medium-sized nitrogen-containing organic molecules, which are the building blocks of proteins. Amino acids are derived from the digestion of dietary protein and reassembled in specific order along templates of RNA, that order being dictated ultimately by DNA.

Anemia Any condition characterized by a decrease in the total body red cell mass.

Anemia of chronic disease The anemia that accompanies general systemic illnesses, especially those characterized by inflammation.

Aplastic anemia The condition characterized by the death of blood cell precursors in the marrow. This results not only in anemia but usually in decreased white cell and platelet counts as well.

B_{12} (vitamin B_{12}) A vitamin that appears to assist folate in the formation of the nucleotide thymidylate. B_{12} has other roles in physiology, such as the breakdown of fats.

Bilirubin A pigmented substance that is the waste product of heme breakdown. The abnormal accumulation of bilirubin in tissues is called jaundice.

Coagulation factors A group of plasma proteins that interact with each other (and with other substances in blood and tissue) to form blood clots.

Cobalamin B_{12}

Cold agglutinin disease An immunohemolytic anemia resulting from autoantibodies that can destroy red cells only at temperatures considerably lower than normal body temperature.

Combined systems disease The progressive deterioration of the brain, spinal cord, and nerves caused by lack of B_{12}.

Cytoplasm The part of a cell that lies within the cell membrane but outside the nucleus. Red cells consist of cytoplasm and cell membrane only.

Direct Coombs test The laboratory test used to make the diagnosis of immunohemolytic anemia. It detects the presence of antibodies coating the patient's red cells.

Disseminated intravascular coagulopathy (DIC) A condition characterized by the formation of tiny clots in blood vessels throughout the body.

DNA Deoxyribonucleic acid, the molecular medium on which the genetic code is inscribed and passed down from one generation to the next. The information in DNA is expressed through the assembly of amino acids into proteins along an RNA template, which is a mediator between DNA and the assembling protein.

Erythroblasts Cells in the bone marrow from which erythrocytes are derived. Unlike the latter, erythroblasts have nuclei.

Erythrocytes Blood cells whose function is the transport of oxygen from the lungs to the rest of the body.

Ferritin A protein that stores iron in various parts of the body, especially the marrow.

Fibrin The protein of which blood clots are composed.

Folate A vitamin necessary for the normal production of the nucleotide thymidylate. Lack of folate causes megaloblastic anemia.

Folic acid Folate.

Globin subunits (or globin chains) The protein molecules that together with heme molecules make up the hemoglobin molecule. The different types of globin subunits are referred to by Greek letters. Thus, the principal hemoglobin of adults (hemoglobin A) is composed of 2 alpha and 2 beta subunits.

Glucose-6-phosphate dehydrogenase (G6PD) An enzyme in red cells that is important for the deactivation of metabolic toxins generated by normal body processes and by exposure to certain drugs and other substances.

Glucose-6-phosphate dehydrogenase deficiency (G6PD deficiency) The genetic condition, inherited on the X chromosome, in which inadequate amounts of G6PD are produced. The result is hemolytic anemia, especially in response to exposure to oxidant drugs and other substances.

Haptoglobin A normal serum protein that binds with hemoglobin spilled from ruptured red cells, allowing the hemoglobin to be captured and recycled.

Hematocrit The volume of red cells in a patient's blood sample, divided by the total volume of the sample. Also called "packed cell volume."

Hematology The medical subspecialty that deals with the diagnosis and treatment of diseases of the blood and blood-forming organs.

Hematopathology The subspecialty of pathology that is concerned with the diagnostic evaluation of the blood and blood-forming organs.

Heme A medium-sized, iron-containing molecule that combines with globin subunits to form hemoglobin.

Hemoglobin 1) A large, complex molecule found exclusively in erythrocytes, the main function of which is the transport of oxygen molecules. Chemically, the hemoglobin molecule consists of 4 smaller protein molecules (globin subunits) and 4 molecules of heme. 2) Shortened form of "hemoglobin concentration in whole blood," one of the cardinal measurements of blood used in clinical hematology.

Hemoglobin A The principal type of hemoglobin in normal people after age 6 months. Hemoglobin A is composed of 2 alpha and 2 beta globin chains.

Hemoglobin C The abnormal form of hemoglobin responsible for hemoglobin C disease. This mutation is seen almost exclusively in persons of African origin. The abnormality affects the beta globin chain.

Hemoglobin concentration in whole blood The mass of hemoglobin per unit volume of a patient's blood.

Hemoglobin E The abnormal form of hemoglobin responsible for hemoglobin E disease. This mutation is seen predominantly in persons of Southeast Asian ancestry. The abnormality affects the beta globin chain.

Hemoglobin F The principal type of hemoglobin in the fetus and young infant. Hemoglobin F is replaced by hemoglobin A by 6 months of age and is composed of 2 alpha and 2 gamma globin chains.

Hemoglobin S The abnormal form of hemoglobin responsible for sickle cell anemia. This mutation is seen predominantly in persons of African and Mediterranean ancestry. The abnormality affects the beta globin chain.

Hemoglobin-oxygen affinity The force with which oxygen is chemically held by hemoglobin molecules. In anemia, the hemoglobin-oxygen affinity decreases to facilitate delivery of oxygen to tissues throughout the body.

Hemoglobinopathy Any genetic condition characterized by an abnormal structure of a globin chain of hemoglobin.

Hemoglobinuria The presence of hemoglobin in the urine.

Hemolysis The abnormal destruction of red blood cells.

Hemolytic anemia An anemia caused by abnormally shortened red cell survival time.

Hemolytic disease of the newborn The immunohemolytic anemia caused by the destruction of a fetus's red cells by its mother's antibodies.

Hereditary spherocytosis The inherited condition in which abnormal structural proteins underneath the red cell's membrane cause the cell to be round instead of biconcave.

Hypochromic A term describing an anemia with a low MCHC (cells with a low concentration of hemoglobin).

Immunohemolytic anemia The hemolytic anemia that occurs as the result of destruction of red cells by antibodies.

Ineffective erythropoiesis The abnormal state characterized by active proliferation of red cell precursors in the marrow but failure of mature red cells to escape into the bloodstream. Ineffective erythropoiesis is an especially prominent feature of thalassemia major and megaloblastic anemia.

Intrinsic factor A substance, produced in the stomach, that combines with B_{12} in the small intestine and allows B_{12} to be absorbed into the body.

Iron A metallic element that is an essential component of heme.

Iron deficiency anemia The microcytic, hypochromic anemia that develops when there is an insufficient amount of iron available to the developing red cells in the marrow.

Leukocytes Blood cells whose main function is to engulf and destroy bacteria and other microorganisms and to modulate the immune response to foreign substances.

Macrocytic A term describing an anemia with a high MCV (large red cells).

MCH Mean corpuscular hemoglobin.

MCHC Mean corpuscular hemoglobin concentration.

MCV Mean corpuscular volume.

Mean corpuscular hemoglobin The average mass of hemoglobin in a patient's red cells.

Mean corpuscular hemoglobin concentration The average concentration of hemoglobin in a patient's red cells.

Mean corpuscular volume The average volume of a patient's red cells, usually measured in femtoliters (fL).

Megaloblastic anemia The anemia that occurs as a result of retarded synthesis of DNA in the developing red cells in the marrow; it is caused by lack of folate and/or B_{12}.

Methyl group A very small organic molecule necessary for the production of the nucleotide thymidylate. Methyl groups can be transferred from one molecule to another only in the presence of folate.

Microangiopathic hemolytic anemia A hemolytic anemia caused by the physical disruption of red cells in the small blood vessels, usually caused by strands of fibrin.

Microcytic A term describing an anemia with a low MCV (small red cells).

Normochromic A term describing an anemia with a normal MCHC (cells have a normal concentration of hemoglobin).

Normocytic A term describing an anemia with a normal MCV (normal-sized red cells).

Nucleotide Any one of 4 medium-sized, nitrogen-containing organic molecules that line up in a specific order to form a molecule of DNA or RNA. The nucleotides that make up DNA are adenylate, thymidylate, cytidylate, and guanylate. RNA is composed of the same 4 nucleotides, except that uridylate takes the place of thymidylate.

Nucleus The part of the cells that contains most (but not all) its genetic information. Red blood cells have no nuclei, but their precursors in the marrow do.

Pernicious anemia The condition that results from failure to absorb vitamin B_{12}, resulting from unavailability of intrinsic factor (IF), resulting from destruction of IF and the cells that produce it.

Pica The craving to eat nonfood substances (e. g., clay, ice, starch). Pica is a symptom of iron deficiency anemia.

Plasma The liquid portion of blood that is not contained within cells (see serum).

Platelets Tiny cell-like structures in the blood, the function of which is to work with the coagulation factors to cause the clotting of blood.

Protein Any one of thousands of different large, complex organic molecules composed of long chains of amino acids assembled in a specific order along a chain-like template of RNA that contains genetic information transcribed from DNA. Proteins have two major functions, serving as (1) structural components of the body, and (2) enzymes, organic catalysts that facilitate many chemical reactions throughout the body.

Red blood cell count The number of red cells in a unit volume of a patient's blood.

Red blood cells (red cells) Erythrocytes

Red cell indices The collective term for 3 important lab measurements in anemia: mean corpuscular volume, mean corpuscular hemoglobin, and mean corpuscular hemoglobin concentration.

Refractory anemia The anemia of unknown cause resulting from damage to blood cell precursors in the marrow, causing ineffective erythropoiesis.

Reticulocyte A young circulating red cell, which can be identified in a specimen by special staining techniques.

Reticuloendothelial system (RES) A widely distributed array of cells, one function of which is the removal of old or damaged blood cells. Cells of the RES are found in the spleen, liver, bone marrow, and lymph nodes.

RNA Ribonucleic acid, the molecular mediator of genetic information between DNA and proteins. RNA is assembled along a DNA template by the process of transcription, and proteins are assembled along the RNA template by the process of translation.

Serum The fluid that remains after plasma is allowed to clot. Serum, then, is plasma, less whatever coagulation factors are consumed in the clotting process.

Sickle cell anemia (or sickle cell disease) The typically severe anemia that results when an individual inherits one gene for hemoglobin S from each parent.

Sickle cell trait The genetic condition that occurs when a person inherits only one sickle cell gene from one parent. Such an individual has no clinical disease.

Thalassemia The inherited condition characterized by the inability to produce sufficient quantities of a structurally normal globin chain. Thalassemias are divided into alpha- and beta-thalassemias, depending on which globin chain is underproduced.

Thalassemia intermedia A form of beta-thalassemia that is not as severe as thalassemia major but may require blood transfusions on occasion.

Thalassemia major The severe, life-threatening form of

beta-thalassemia that requires lifelong transfusions and chelation therapy.

Thalassemia minor   A clinically inconsequential form of beta-thalassemia that causes microcytosis and a mild degree of anemia. It does not require treatment.

Thrombotic thrombocytopenic purpura (TTP)   A condition similar to disseminated intravascular coagulopathy, in which platelets are consumed, but coagulation proteins are not.

Total iron binding capacity   A lab test that measures the amount of transferrin in serum.

Transcription   The process by which the genetic information on DNA is transferred to messenger RNA.

Transferrin   A protein, found in normal serum, that transports iron to the marrow.

Translation   The process by which genetic information in messenger RNA is expressed in the assembly of amino acids to make proteins.

Urobilinogen   A colorless substance that is the result of breakdown of bilirubin by bacteria in the intestines.

Warm autoimmune hemolytic anemia   The immunohemolytic anemia resulting from autoantibodies that are capable of destroying red cells at normal body temperature.

White blood cells (white cells)   Leukocytes.

Wright stain   A commonly used stain for the routine examination of blood cells in the clinical laboratory.

Index